THERE IS NO PERFECT DENTIST

*The Never Berfore Revealed
Secrets to Choosing the*
RIGHT *Dentist for* YOU!

DR. NEIL GERRARD, B.D.S.

NEW YORK

THERE IS NO PERFECT DENTIST

The Never Berfore Revealed Secrets to
Choosing the RIGHT *Dentist for* YOU!

by Dr. Neil Gerrard, B.D.S.

© 2010 Dr. Neil Gerrard, B.D.S. All rights reserved.

No part of this publication may be reproduced or transmitted in any form or by any means, mechanical or electronic, including photocopying and recording, or by any information storage and retrieval system, without permission in writing from author or publisher (except by a reviewer, who may quote brief passages and/or show brief video clips in a review).

Disclaimer: The Publisher and the Author make no representations or warranties with respect to the accuracy or completeness of the contents of this work and specifically disclaim all warranties, including without limitation warranties of fitness for a particular purpose. No warranty may be created or extended by sales or promotional materials. The advice and strategies contained herein may not be suitable for every situation. This work is sold with the understanding that the Publisher is not engaged in rendering legal, accounting, or other professional services. If professional assistance is required, the services of a competent professional person should be sought. Neither the Publisher nor the Author shall be liable for damages arising herefrom. The fact that an organization or website is referred to in this work as a citation and/or a potential source of further information does not mean that the Author or the Publisher endorses the information the organization or website may provide or recommendations it may make. Further, readers should be aware that internet websites listed in this work may have changed or disappeared between when this work was written and when it is read.

ISBN 978-0-98285-900-1 (paperback)
Library of Congress Control Number: 2010931846

Published by:

GLAZER KENNEDY PUBLISHING
an imprint of Morgan James Publishing
1225 Franklin Ave. Ste 325
Garden City, NY 11530-1693
Toll Free 800-485-4943
www.MorganJamesPublishing.com

Cover Design by:
Rachel Lozez
rachel@r2cdesign.com

Interior Design by:
Bonnie Bushman
bbushman@bresnan.net

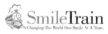

Smile Train is dedicated to funding free cleft lip and palate surgery for millions of poor children in developing countries worldwide, while providing free cleft related training for doctors and medical professionals. Dr. Neil Gerrard and There is no Perfect Dentist proudly support the work of Smile Train, donating 25 percent of all royalties from the sale of each book to this worthy cause.

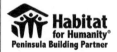

In an effort to support local communities, raise awareness and funds, Morgan James Publishing donates one percent of all book sales for the life of each book to Habitat for Humanity. Get involved today, visit
www.HelpHabitatForHumanity.org.

ACKNOWLEDGEMENTS

I wish to thank the following people for their valued support and advice in the publication of this book:

Mrs Stephanie Burton, Clinical Hypnotherapist EDH, DHP, MNCH (Reg.)

Dr. John Chope, BDS, BSc Brist., RCS Eng., DGDP (UK), LDS

Dr. Lester Ellman, BDS

Dr. Alan Holland, MSc Lond., BChD Leeds, LDS RCS Eng

Dr. Elliot Mechanic BSc, DDS

Dr. Bertrand Napier, BDS (Rand.)

Dr. Tom Orent, DDS

Dr. Christopher Orr, BDS, BSc

My final thank you is dedicated to my wife Fiona for her support, patience and understanding, for without which this book would not have been possible.

TABLE OF CONTENTS

Acknowledgements		iii
Introduction		vii
Professional Obligation		xi

PART ONE: COSMETIC DENTISTRY — 1

1	What's the Difference Between Cosmetic and Aesthetic Dentistry?	3
2	What Type of People Choose Cosmetic Dentistry?	5
3	What You Should Consider Before Starting Treatment	7
4	What types of smiles are suitable for treatment?	9
5	Why Do People Say No to Cosmetic Dentistry?	13

PART TWO: HOW TO CHOOSE YOUR PERFECT DENTIST — 17

6	Fifteen Questions You Must Ask When Choosing a Dentist	19
7	Where to Look When Searching for Your Perfect Dentist	29
8	What Your Dentist Should Do Next	35
9	Dental Tourism—What You Must Know before Considering Treatment Abroad	39

PART THREE: THE NHS, PRIVATE DENTAL CARE, AND DENTAL HEALTH INSURANCE — 45

10	The National Health Service (NHS)	47
11	Five Reasons to Consider Private Dentistry	51
12	The Cost of a Healthy Mouth and Smile	55

13 Dental Health Insurance   59

PART FOUR: DEFEATING FEAR OF
THE DENTIST   63

14 Five Ways to Defeat Fear of the Dentist   65
15 Distraction Techniques   67
16 Desensitisation Therapy   69
17 Hypnotherapy   71
18 Cognitive Behavioral Therapy (CBT)   73
19 Use of Medication and Dental Sedation   75

PART FIVE: ROLE OF THE SPECIALIST
AND DENTAL TEAM   81

20 Why You May Consider the Help of a Specialist to
    Transform Your Smile or Dental Health   83
21 Dental Care Professionals (DCPs)—Who Are They and
    What Do They Do?   99
22 What Do the Letters Stand For?   105

PART SIX: RESOLVING PROBLEMS   109

23 What if Things Go Wrong?   111
24 Complications Following Treatment   113
25 Communication   115
26 Treatment Charges   117
27 Handling of Complaints   119
28 Local Resolution   123
29 Dental Complaints Service   125
30 NHS Complaints Service   127
31 The GDC (General Dental Council)   131
32 Take Legal Action—a Word of Warning!   133

PART SEVEN: FREE AUDIO, CONTACTS
AND GLOSSARY   137

33 **FREE** Audio Recording and special report   139
34 Useful Contacts   141
35 Glossary of Terms   145

INTRODUCTION

It's unsurprising that many people struggle to find the perfect dentist. The choices we face as consumers in today's society can be overwhelming, whether purchasing any product or seeking dental care. Not only are we faced with a diverse range of choices, but many of the messages conveyed to us can appear to offer conflicting information, thus making our decisions even more confusing.

When considering a new dentist or a particular treatment, a myriad of choices present themselves. Decisions must be made, including: the type of treatment required, quality of care required, your budget, private versus NHS care, and finally the dentist him or herself.

Choosing a dentist was described to me by one colleague as, "like choosing an electrician or plumber." If you find a "good one," then great; if not, you may find yourself regretting it later. So, how do you find a "good one," a dentist you not only like and trust but who is also able to provide the type of care you are looking for? When there is no such thing as the perfect dentist for everyone, how do you choose the perfect dentist for you? These are the questions I have attempted to answer within this book.

As an accredited member and examiner for the British Academy of Cosmetic Dentistry (BACD), I have improved the lives and health of hundreds of patients who have come to me for help, people who have found me to be the perfect dentist for them. With a little help, I believe it is possible for anyone interested in doing so to find the perfect dentist as well.

Because of my special interest in cosmetic dentistry, many of my recommendations throughout the book refer to cosmetic dentistry as illustrations. Cosmetic dentists must be skilled in the creation of new smiles, but they must also possess the skills to complete quality general dental care (as this is the foundation for many cosmetic procedures). So, whether you are interested in improving the appearance of your smile, replacing missing or broken teeth, or simply improving the general health of your teeth and gums, my recommendations are relevant to all.

Until the widespread introduction and use of the Internet, the only way to choose a dentist was to either seek recommendations from friends and family or to look in the yellow pages. Nowadays quality information is readily available online. However, much of this is directed toward the types of treatments available and what they involve. Up until now, unbiased information offering advice on how to choose the right dentist for you has been lacking. This book is aimed at addressing this disparity.

If you are unhappy with your smile, if you would like to find out more about your options, or if you have already decided to improve your smile or dental health but don't know where to start, then reading this book is an excellent starting point.

The information contained within these pages is designed to provide knowledge—knowledge required to make one of the most important decisions you will ever make as you ask yourself: How would I like to smile? Do I want to improve my dental health? Where do I go and who do I ask to fix it?

About the Structure of This Book

For ease of reading and quick reference to relevant information, this book is divided into seven parts.

> **Part One** discusses cosmetic dentistry, who is suitable for treatment, and why to consider it.
>
> **Part Two** tells you how to choose the perfect dentist for you, where to look, and what you should expect from your first visit.
>
> **Part Three** discuses NHS and private dental care—including dental health insurance.

Part Four will help you overcome fear of the dentist.

Part Five discusses the role of the dental specialist and the dental team.

Part Six will help you deal with problems and disagreements.

Part Seven offers useful contacts and a glossary of terminology.

PROFESSIONAL OBLIGATION

As a registered dentist, I must be careful to comply with the rules set by my professional governing body, the General Dental Council (GDC). It is a legal requirement that all practicing dentists within the UK must be registered with the GDC if they wish to treat patients.

The GDC stipulates that no registered dentist can claim or imply to be better than another, neither can he or she publicly criticise a fellow colleague's work or standard of clinical care. Breaking these rules is considered unprofessional and can result in termination of a dentist's registration.

This book will therefore offer no preference of any one dental professional's services above that of another. Its sole aim is to provide knowledge and impartial advice.

Throughout this book, you will see reference to a number of Internet services where you can locate your perfect dentist. In the interest of disclosure and maintaining an unbiased position, I declare that I hold a personal and financial interest in one such service, *www. MyPerfectDentist.com.*

As a member of the public, you can obtain additional information from the General Dental Council (GDC) at *www.gdc-uk.org.* The GDC holds a list of all registered dentists and dental care professionals (DCPs) in the UK.

PART ONE

COSMETIC DENTISTRY

1

What's the Difference Between Cosmetic and Aesthetic Dentistry?

Cosmetic dentistry is a term widely used by the media, general public, and dentists to describe a range of treatments aimed at altering the appearance of an individual's smile.

Treatments most often thought of as cosmetic in nature are porcelain laminate veneers, crowns, bridges, and tooth-whitening procedures, but other treatments may also possesses a cosmetic component, which include: the replacement of missing or damaged teeth with dental implants, placement of direct composite (white) fillings or artistic bonding, orthodontic treatments, and even the use of removable dentures.

When considering and researching these types of treatments, you will probably encounter the term aesthetic dentistry. This is a term used infrequently by the media or general public but widely within the dental profession. It is therefore important that you understand the distinct difference between the two, as this may affect your choice of treatment or even dentist.

In this context, the term *cosmetic dentistry* best describes the anatomy of a tooth or smile modified in such a way as to produce an appearance very pleasing to the eye but enhanced beyond what is normally found in nature—an enhanced natural appearance.

However, the term *aesthetic dentistry* best describes the anatomy of a tooth or smile modified in such a way to replicate nature and all its intricacies to the last detail or the reproduction of a natural smile as nature intended.

Most dentists will use these terms interchangeably to refer to any treatment that involves the repair, replacement, or improvement of a tooth or smile, whether enhanced beyond that which nature intended (cosmetic) or conforming to an existing natural appearance (aesthetic).

However, some dentists make a point of stating they perform aesthetic dentistry in preference to cosmetic dentistry. This does not mean they do not offer the full range of cosmetic procedures as you would understand them (just as a cosmetic dentist will offer aesthetic dentistry when requested), but that they have chosen to distinguish the difference between the two out of personal preference and philosophy of care.

In reality, the most attractive smiles are those created by mother-nature, which in turn are copied by cosmetic/aesthetic dentists. By using those natural features scientifically proven to be most attractive to the human eye, both cosmetic and aesthetic dentists can recreate the most beautifully natural smiles, or the brightest, widest enhanced smiles aspired to by many in today's society.

For the purpose of this book, I have used the term cosmetic dentistry to describe any procedure associated with the alteration of a smile.

2
WHAT TYPE OF PEOPLE CHOOSE COSMETIC DENTISTRY?

I have helped improve the lives of men and women of all ages and from all walks of life, from celebrities and high-flying business executives to shop assistants and waitresses.

What do all these people have in common, and why did they decide to seek cosmetic dentistry?

What made these people seek cosmetic dentistry were the same feelings of self-consciousness and embarrassment when smiling that you probably feel right now. They all wanted to feel more attractive, more confident, and more relaxed in their professional and personal lives.

For example:

Both Trudy and David came to me for help with their upcoming weddings. One a bank clerk, the other a wealthy director of a national company, both of them self-conscious about smiling in photographs, both wanting to enjoy their weddings without fear of the camera, both wanting to avoid wedding photos that would haunt them for years to come.

Further examples are Louise, a finance administrator, and Paul, a computer engineer. Both were tired of feeling inadequate, and both were tired of hiding their smiles from customers and colleagues at work. They both wanted to feel confident, they both wanted to feel good about their smiles, and they both wanted to eliminate the dread of smiling once and for all.

Just imagine how Trudy, David, Paul, and Louise felt once they underwent cosmetic dentistry to improve their smiles—self-assured and attractive.

I have many more stories just like theirs of everyday people all wanting to feel great about their smiles. You can read more about the people who have made the decision to smile with confidence by visiting, *www.CliftonSmiles.com* or many other dental-related Web sites.

No matter who you are, what problems you have, or how bad you feel about your smile, cosmetic dentistry can help. There is virtually no smile that cannot be improved, no problem too big or small that cannot be overcome with cosmetic dentistry.

3

WHAT YOU SHOULD CONSIDER BEFORE STARTING TREATMENT

Demand for cosmetic and private dentistry has grown significantly in the past ten years, with the British public now spending around 3 billion pounds per year on private dentistry, of which nearly 1 billion pounds is spent specifically on cosmetic dental procedures.[1]

Regardless of the popularity of cosmetic dentistry in today's society and all of the positive benefits it offers, I feel it is important that you understand both the positive as well as the negative implications of both cosmetic and general dental treatments.

Cosmetic dentistry offers an invaluable service to people; it literally changes lives. People once embarrassed or even fearful to smile in public find themselves with a newfound confidence they never expected in both their personal and professional relationships. But as with many things in life, there is a compromise to be had. The obvious positive benefits of a great-looking, confident smile must always be balanced against a small number of negative aspects associated with some dental procedures.

Whenever a tooth is treated (whether a diseased tooth or for cosmetic enhancement), it inevitably requires the removal of healthy tooth enamel. Virtually all fillings, veneers, crowns, and bridges require removal of healthy tooth enamel to succeed, both functionally and

---

1 Figures supplied courtesy of the British Dental Association (BDA).

aesthetically. Now, this would be of little consequence except for one problem. Dentists have yet to develop a filling/veneer/crown material that not only looks exactly like a tooth but functions like a tooth as well. There is no man-made material that will last as long as your own tooth (a lifetime), which means at some point in time it is likely that your new filling, crown, or cosmetically enhanced smile will wear out and require replacement.

So, of what relevance is this to you?

If your smile is worn out, has been heavily treated in the past, or you possess multiple missing teeth, then this will probably be of little relevance. If your smile has already reached this point, then the benefits of treatment will far outweigh any need for future care, as future care is already a necessity.

However, if you possess pristine, perfectly healthy teeth and you are twenty years of age, then the idea of removing healthy tooth enamel is probably not in your best long-term interest. It is likely that if left untreated, your teeth will last for decades to come, in fact significantly longer than any filling or veneer when looked after correctly.

Scientific research[2] indicates that the average life expectancy of porcelain veneers, crowns, and bridges is around ten to fifteen years, so when considering treatment, you must accept that once you commit to a procedure, you will need to undertake that procedure again, maybe once, twice, or even three times over your lifetime. Common sense dictates that the greater the loss of healthy tooth enamel now, the less will be available to treat later. You may even reach a point at which so little tooth remains that re-treatment is no longer an option.

When considering any cosmetic dental procedure, my advice is always the same: first, make sure you have all the information you require to make an informed choice, and second, consider both the benefits and disadvantages of a procedure before undertaking treatment. There is no right or wrong answer, just what is right for you.

---

2   Fradeani M, et al. "Porcelain Laminate Veneers 6- to 12-year Clinical Evaluation—A Retrospective Study." *International Journal of Periodontics & Restorative Dentistry.* 2005; 25:9-17.

Friedman M.J. "A 15 Year Review of Porcelain Veneer Failure—A Clinician's Observations." *Compen Contin Educ Dent.* 1998; 19:625-632.

4

WHAT TYPES OF SMILES ARE SUITABLE FOR TREATMENT?

Advancements in dentistry have now reached a point at which virtually anyone can be helped. Whether you wish to improve the size, shape, colour, or position of your teeth and smile, or just chew in comfort, dentistry offers a number of solutions. For the majority of people the only limiting factor is the willingness to complete those treatments necessary to reach their desired goals.

What should your existing smile look like for maximum benefit?

To the vast majority of people, the term "cosmetic dentistry" involves the enhancement of a smile with porcelain veneers, crowns, and bridges.

Those individuals most suited to this type of treatment are those possessing teeth that are worn, heavily filled, or missing. Basically, if there is any starting point that we dentists can add to, rather than subtract from. For example, when teeth are heavily worn or filled, porcelain veneers can be built up over the existing tooth enamel with little or no reduction of healthy tooth structure (it has already worn away). However, when teeth possess little or no wear, healthy tooth enamel must be reduced to make room for the veneers, and in some cases very aggressive reduction is required.

Smiles that benefit most from these "cosmetic treatments" include those with:

- Tooth wear (intermediate to severe)
- Missing teeth
- Diseased teeth
- Developmental tooth defects
- Tooth loss/damaged through trauma
- Gaps—due to small teeth or excess space
- Discoloured teeth
- Bite problems

People of all ages may benefit from this additive approach. The young may possess congenitally missing teeth (teeth that never developed), developmental tooth defects (weak, thin, or missing tooth enamel), small or spaced teeth, or they may have lost teeth through trauma (accidental damage). The middle aged and elderly may possess missing, very worn, and heavily filled teeth. These are all situations that lend themselves well to cosmetic enhancement without the need to excessively reduce previously healthy tooth enamel, as wear and tear has already occurred.

Smiles that meet this type of pre-treatment criteria allow conservative treatment options to be used, treatments that require either minimal or even no enamel removal from a tooth in order to improve its appearance and function.

What if your smile meets none of these criteria?

If your smile meets none of these criteria, it doesn't mean you cannot or should not improve your smile. It just means that alternative solutions may offer a great result without the need for tooth reduction and a subsequent lifetime commitment to dental treatments in years to come.

Smiles that benefit most from these "alternative" treatment approaches are those requiring no enamel reduction, otherwise perfectly healthy smiles possessing:

- Crooked or twisted teeth
- Very young teeth—those typically under twenty to twenty-five years of age
- Gaps
- Crowded teeth
- Discolored teeth
- Bite problems

Smiles meeting these types of pre-treatment criteria are often most suited to enhancement with orthodontic treatments (braces), direct composite bonding (artistic bonding), and tooth-whitening treatments if the aim is long-term health and wellbeing.

What treatments should you consider if your smile falls between these two groups or you are determined to undertake "cosmetic dentistry"?

There will always be individuals with smiles that fall between the very worn, damaged, or missing teeth and the perfectly healthy but crooked smile, just as there will always be individuals who feel they must own the perfect "Hollywood" smile.

Under these circumstances, I would always advise you to consider a multi-disciplinary treatment approach (treatment that employs a number of different treatment methods to reach your desired goals). For example, if your teeth are perfectly healthy but crooked and you want the brighter whiter "Hollywood smile," then an excellent way forward is to straighten your existing smile with orthodontics, followed by tooth whitening. If you still feel your smile would benefit from porcelain veneers following this, then you are in the perfect position to take advantage of veneers requiring the most conservative enamel removal, or no enamel removal at all, rather than the most aggressive.

Further information regarding all types of dental treatments and what they involve can be easily sourced online, or through sites like *www.MyPerfectDentist.com* and *www.CosmeticDentistryGuide.com*.

5

WHY DO PEOPLE SAY NO TO COSMETIC DENTISTRY?

After considering the improvement of their smiles, why do some people decide not to proceed with cosmetic dentistry? Why, when they feel so uncomfortable with their smiles, do they decide to do nothing? Why? Because of many reasons, but the main ones are:

- They just can't decide if treatment is right for them
- Fear of the unknown
- Fear of painful treatment
- They cannot find a "good" cosmetic dentist
- They decide it is too expensive

They Just Can't Decide if Treatment Is Right for Them

Are you truly unhappy with your smile? If so, then this first reason is not relevant, but some people decide cosmetic dentistry is not for them because they do not realize how good a new smile will make them feel. They do not realize how truly unhappy they are and will continue to hide their smiles despite the many benefits a new smile can offer. They just cannot imagine the way a great smile can literally change lives.

Studies[3] indicate that the mouth is responsible for *60 to 70 percent* of the visual perception of the face, meaning this is what we notice most consciously and subconsciously when interacting with other people. This

3 Data supplied by Dr. Elliot Mechanic BSc., DDS. 1 Place du commerce, suite 100, Montreal, Quebec, Canada H3E 1A3.

13

knowledge alone should be a big enough reason to improve your smile, let alone the lack of confidence that warrants a change in your life.

Why do you think that every person chosen for the makeover shows on television like *Ten Years Younger* and *Extreme Makeover* have their smiles fixed? Because no face-lift, eyebrow lift, jowl lift, facial skin peel, or Botox® can change a person's appearance as drastically as a brilliant new smile.

Please ask yourself, do you want the smile you have always dreamed of, or do you want a smile you are ashamed of? If you want a dream smile, then cosmetic dentistry may be right for you.

Fear of the Unknown

Fear of the unknown is only natural, and some people panic so much about how they will look afterward that they just cannot bring themselves to undertake treatment.

I have personally experienced treatment as an adult with fixed "tram-track" braces, and I was naturally concerned about how I would look, so I understand exactly how you feel. The great news is that modern cosmetic dentistry now enables you to see your new smile before you even start, so there really is no need to panic!

Most experienced cosmetic dentists can help you see your smile's potential before you make the decision to change it. It is now possible to preview your new smile in a number of ways. For example:

Computer imaging of you in a photo, producing a realistic before and after photo of your new smile

A mock-up on a 3D model—a real model of your teeth you can pick up and look at from every angle

A direct mock-up of your new smile in your mouth—simulated stick on veneers placed in just a few minutes so you can see the results (without changing your teeth in any way)

What about During Treatment?

In most cases, a trial-smile will be placed on your teeth during treatment. This enables you to test-drive your new smile before it is finished, offering you the opportunity to check the size, shape, and colour of your new teeth.

If you do not like it, you can change it and continue to alter it until you are completely happy. Once satisfied, your trial smile is used as a template from which your new smile is copied, so you have a good idea what to expect when your smile is completed.

Fear of Painful Treatment

Admittedly, we dentists do not have the best reputation when it comes to dental treatment. We are generally known for delivering an uncomfortable and painful experience.

This should no longer be the case. Modern state-of-the-art dentistry is not an agonising experience. *In expert hands, you will experience relaxed treatment, with minimal or no discomfort at all.*

Even the most nervous of patients can now achieve the smile of his or her dreams with dental sedation. This stuff is truly impressive; you will not have a care in the world, and treatment will pass by in what feels like minutes. In fact, you may even enjoy it! There really is no reason to be fearful anymore.

What About After Treatment?

You are probably asking, what about afterward? Sure, for a couple of days after treatment you may feel a little bruised, but nothing that over-the-counter painkillers can't control.

I personally suffer from a long-term back problem resulting from a car crash, for which I regularly visit an osteopath for treatment. I can be sore for a couple of days after each visit, but the benefits of treatment far outweigh any short-term discomfort.

This is exactly the same as improving your smile. If you have never been able to smile with confidence, it is difficult to imagine how you will feel after cosmetic dentistry, but believe me, the feeling you will experience the first time you smile is nothing short of life changing.

They Cannot Find a "Good" Cosmetic Dentist

Placing your smile in the hands of a total stranger takes trust. You need to feel certain that the dentist you have chosen understands what you want and that as a professional he or she possesses the necessary skills to make it a reality.

Finding the right cosmetic dentist can take time and effort, but again, the rewards far outweigh the inconvenience of having to read up on the subject.

Asking friends or family is no longer your only option. Books and reports like this one, or Web services like *www.MyPerfectDentist.com,* now allow you to find the information you really need to make an informed choice.

They Decide It Is Too Expensive

We have all heard stories of Hollywood movie stars spending hundreds of thousands of pounds on their smiles and face-lifts, but such spending is not always necessary. In reality, it is possible to improve your smile with a range of less-expensive treatments. For example, tooth whitening, a treatment that generally starts from just a few hundred pounds, may be all that is needed to rejuvenate your smile.

If you are considering a smile makeover or porcelain veneers, then yes, cosmetic dentistry can be costly. I have treated some very wealthy people who did not need to consider the cost of anything, whether it be a holiday, new car, or a confident new smile. For most of us, however, cost is a consideration. That is why most cosmetic dentists offer a range of treatments to meet most needs and to suit most budgets. Many practitioners offer a number of ways to make payment affordable, like interest-free credit or monthly payment plans. Cosmetic dentistry has made great strides toward affordability.

When considering cost, my advice is always the same. Pay for the best quality you can possibly afford from the most experienced dentist you kind find. Remember, this is your smile, and it is priceless.

PART TWO

HOW TO CHOOSE YOUR PERFECT DENTIST

6

FIFTEEN QUESTIONS YOU MUST ASK WHEN CHOOSING A DENTIST

What should you look for when seeking your ideal dentist? What should you be asking yourself when reading brochures and Web sites or receiving a recommendation? What questions should you ask the dentist and their staff?

The first thing you must do is know the right questions to ask. As an experienced cosmetic dentist, these are the questions I would ask if I were seeking cosmetic or general dentistry.

1. **Is the Dentist Registered with the General Dental Council (GDC)?**

   Every year a small number of people are found guilty of practicing dentistry illegally—either pretending to be a dentist or having previously been a dentist and are now removed from the dental register for substandard treatment, fraud, or unethical behaviour. You do not want to place your smile and dental well-being in the hands of these people!

   You can easily check whether your chosen dentist is registered to legally practice in the UK by visiting the GDC online at *www.gdc-uk.org*. Alternatively, you can ask the dentist and their staff to present their registration certificates.

2. **Does the Dentist Have a Special Interest in Any Particular Field of Dentistry?**

    Why should you ask this? There is no such specialist qualification in cosmetic or implant dentistry like orthodontics or oral surgery. Any dentist can legally state that he holds a special interest in a particular field if he predominantly practices that type of dentistry and has completed extensive training to support this.

    Many of the best dentists in the country have a special interest in cosmetic and implant dentistry. They have completed hundreds of hours of training in cosmetic procedures and spend most of their time providing cosmetic and dental implant treatments.

    If a dentist states that he or she has a special interest in cosmetic dentistry but treats just a handful of patients per year, then it is likely he or she is spending most of his or her time on other treatments, such as basic fillings or removing teeth.

3. **What Types of Treatment Does the Dentist Offer?**

    This sounds like a silly question, doesn't it? What type of treatment does the cosmetic dentist provide? It is actually a very important question.

    Most cosmetic dentists provide a similar range of treatments, such as porcelain veneers and crowns. However, the quality and appearance of these will vary significantly from the most beautiful to the very average.

    What you should be looking for is the telltale signs that distinguish the very best from the very average. In the case of cosmetic dentistry, one effective trick is to ask the dentist if he offers *direct* bonding and *directly* bonded veneers.

    These are treatments created solely by the dentist without the help of a dental technician. Performing this treatment well requires tremendous skill and a commitment to learning. If the dentist is capable of producing the most beautiful smiles in this way, he should be capable of providing the very best smiles no matter what type of treatment is required.

4. **Does the Dentist Have Before and After Photos of Real People He or She Has Actually Treated?**

You may be surprised by the answer. Very often, cosmetic dentists provide "stock" photos showing the results of *other dentists'* work. A shocker–and a sign you need to look elsewhere. After all, cosmetic dentists who are really good—and proud of their skill—don't need to show you some stranger's work. They are happy to show their own.

A first-rate, experienced cosmetic dentist will be delighted to show you before and after photos of patients he or she has actually treated. The mere fact that photos of real patients are available is a testament to how thrilled they feel about their new smiles; otherwise, they would never have allowed the dentist to show them.

5. **How Many *Cases* Like Yours Has the Dentist Completed?**

Why did I put emphasis on the word *cases*? Because it's the magic word if you want an answer that really means something.

Ask a dentist how many veneers he has done and he may answer perfectly honestly and say 120. While it sounds like a tremendous amount of experience, it could simply mean he's done roughly ten teeth each for just twelve patients. Ask how many veneer cases he's done and he will say twelve—not a terrible number, but nowhere nearly as reassuring as 120!

The number of cases the dentist has done is one important way to judge his experience, but there are other ways to determine level of experience as well.

6. **How Many Years Has He or She Been Performing the Procedure?**

As I'm sure you could guess for yourself, longer is better—for two reasons. You want a dentist who is highly experienced, and a dentist who has been doing a procedure for five or ten years knows for sure that his work stands the test of time.

7. **Does He or She Have Testimonials from Other Grateful Patients?**

You want to know what people like you have to say about the dentist's work. Are patients totally delighted with the results? Do they love the way they look? Do they smile more, laugh more, and feel more comfortable and outgoing?

Take your time and read their stories carefully. You want to see for yourself how much the dentist's work has meant to other people.

Don't stop there, though. As I'm sure you know, no dentist would show letters from unhappy patients, so you want to get beyond the people who were so thrilled they simply had to write to say thank you. You also want to talk to folks who haven't written.

Maybe they thanked the dentist in person. Maybe they just aren't the letter writing type. Or maybe—just maybe—they were unhappy about the work the dentist did. You'll never know if you don't ask. Ask if he has any patients who would not mind talking to you about their experiences. When you talk to these patients, don't hold back. Ask about anything and everything that might concern you. Find out exactly what the dentist did and how the patient likes the result. Ask about how long it took and how comfortable (or uncomfortable) the procedure was. Find out if the patient feels that the work has made a real difference in his or her life.

8. **Is the Dentist an Active Member of a Professional Association that Represents His or Her Area of Expertise and Special Interest?**

Each field of dentistry is normally represented by its own association. Two examples of specialist associations are the British Society of Periodontology (gum specialists) and the

British Orthodontic Society (specialists in braces). These associations represent and help educate dentists in their field of expertise.

If seeking a cosmetic dentist, ask if the dentist is a member of at least one of these associations: BACD (The British Academy of Cosmetic Dentistry), BAAD (The British Academy of Aesthetic Dentistry), or AACD (The American Academy of Cosmetic Dentistry).

If you are seeking a dentist offering dental implants, you should ask if he is a member of the ADI (Association of Dental Implantology), ICOI (The International Congress of Oral Implantologists), or EAO (European Association for Osseointegration).

The British Academy of Cosmetic Dentistry (BACD) is the largest organisation in the UK dedicated to the art and science of cosmetic dentistry. Further information can be found at *www.bacd.com.* Associations also dedicated to cosmetic dentistry are The American Academy of Cosmetic Dentistry (AACD), at *www.aacd.com,* and The British Academy of Aesthetic Dentistry (BAAD), at *www.baad.org.uk.*

9. **Does the Dentist Possess Any Formal Records of Achievement from the Association that Represents His or Her Area of Expertise?**

If you are choosing a cosmetic dentist, ask the dentist if he is an accredited member of the BACD or AACD. Both the British Academy of Cosmetic Dentistry (BACD) and American Academy of Cosmetic Dentistry (AACD) provide a credentialing pathway designed to test and examine their member dentists' skills and knowledge in the field of cosmetic dentistry.

Accreditation represents an ability to provide the very best smiles and the highest standard of care in the field of cosmetic dentistry. At the time of publication, only eight dentists in the UK have achieved such recognition with the BACD.

This type of credentialing pathway is not limited to cosmetic dentistry alone. A number of associations representing other areas of interest also offer similar peer assessments, recognising the skills and commitment of their member dentists (e.g., implant dentistry).

10. **Does the Dentist Regularly Take Continuing Education Courses to Stay Up-to-Date with the Latest Techniques in Clinical Cosmetic Dentistry?**

It is a statutory registration requirement with the General Dental Council (GDC) that all dentists undertake a minimum of 250 hours of continuing education every five years (average fifty hours per year). This requirement is intended to maintain professional standards of care and so protect the general public.

This is extremely important. Both private and NHS dental practices are not large hospitals. Doctors working in hospitals have the opportunity to discuss the best treatments for their patients and seek second opinions from fellow doctors every day. As a dentist working alone in practice, I have no one to confer with. The only way I can offer my patients the best possible care and keep up-to-date with the latest procedures (in both cosmetic and general dentistry) is to undertake many hours of continuing education in the UK, Europe, and America.

To join and remain a member of an association like the BACD, a dentist must complete at least twenty-five hours of recognised training per year in the field of cosmetic dentistry.

The very best cosmetic and general dentists will complete many more hours of training per year than the minimum fifty hours average required by the GDC.

This level of commitment is another way of separating the very best from the average.

11. **Does the Dentist Teach Other Members of the Profession?**

Some dentists are actively involved in the education of other dental professionals.

To do so often requires extensive practical expertise and an excellent understanding of the latest research and best practice. The result, that many are leaders in their fields of interest.

Choosing to undertake treatment with a dentist involved in the education of others can be another way of seeking those offering the very best care.

12. **Is a Guarantee on Treatment Offered, and if so, What Does It Cover and for How Long?**

For peace of mind, many dentists will offer some form of consumer protection against prematurely failing treatment— for example, a promise to replace any porcelain veneer and crown at no cost if it fails within five years of treatment.

Why do the best dentists offer this? They offer this because they are confident that their treatments will not only look good but also last the test of time. If you are seriously considering cosmetic dentistry or even routine dental treatment, a comprehensive policy against failure is another indication of a dentist's competency in providing the very best long-lasting care.

It is important to note that as a patient you will be expected to meet a number of conditions for any such offer to remain valid, e.g. all necessary dental care must be completed, while regular dental health examinations and maintenance care must be undertaken.

When researching guarantees, you are likely to find small print appearing to absolve dentists of any responsibility, with phrases like promise and policy used in place of the word guarantee. Don't be put you off!

Guarantee is a term that possesses a specific legal definition in consumer law not easily applied to living beings. If you are unsure what these promises or policies actually mean, ask for written confirmation before undertaking treatment.

13. **Has the Dentist's Staff, or Any of Their Family Members, Had Cosmetic Work Done by the Dentist?**

Obviously, if the staff hasn't asked the dentist to work on them, then you probably don't want to either. And if they have had work done by the dentist, you'll have the chance to get a "live" look at what he can do.

14. **Which Dental Technician or Laboratory Does the Dentist Use if You Are Undertaking Treatment for Porcelain Veneers, Crowns, or Implants?**

Many laboratories and technicians create the veneers and crowns dentists use on a daily basis to restore or improve the appearance of an individual's teeth and smile. As with dentists, there can be a significant difference in the technician's abilities and skill, ranging from average to the very best.

Knowing which technician and laboratory your dentist works with to create his crowns and veneers will offer you the opportunity to research them. (Information can normally be sourced on the Web with little effort.) As a layman, the easiest method for determining a good dental technician is to see what he charges for his services. As a guide in 2010, the average fee for quality produced veneers and crowns can range from £150 to around £250 per tooth. When browsing the Web, you will likely find some technicians charging as little as £21.00 or less for a single crown, while others may charge up to £600.

Choosing a dentist who works with a quality technician or laboratory is a good indication that you have chosen a conscientious dentist with high standards of clinical care.

15. **What Does the Dentist Charge for Treatments?**

When considering any dental treatment, you should never look for the cheapest. There is no such thing as a free lunch, and when it comes to most dental treatments, the old adage "you get what you pay for" has never been truer.

There will always be a variation in what each dentist charges for a particular procedure. Porcelain veneers, crowns, and dental implants are not commodities, but bespoke items. As such, each dentist will set his or her fees at a level representing his or her skill and experience, the quality of care provided, and the costs of running a private dental practice.

One other important note—do not make the mistake of thinking that what you are paying for is a veneer, crown, dental implant, or even a filling. You obviously are, but what you are truly paying for is the dentist's knowledge. The greater his knowledge and experience, the better quality the final results, whether it is treatment with braces, dental implants, cosmetic dental procedures, or a standard filling.

To Summarise:

- Is the dentist registered with the General Dental Council (GDC)?

- Does the dentist have a special interest in any particular field of dentistry?

- What types of treatment does the dentist offer?

- Does the dentist have before and after photos of real people he or she has actually treated?

- How many *cases* like yours has the dentist completed?

- How many years has he or she been performing the procedure?

- Does he or she have testimonials from other grateful patients?

- Is the dentist an active member of a professional association that represents his or her area of expertise and special interest?

- Does the dentist possess any formal records of achievement from the association that represents his or her area of expertise?

- Does the dentist regularly take continuing education courses to stay up-to-date with the latest techniques in his or her area of expertise?

- Does the dentist teach other members of the profession?

- Is a guarantee on treatment offered, and if so, what does it cover and for how long?

- Has the dentist's staff, or any of their family members, had cosmetic work done by the dentist?

- Which dental technician or laboratory does the dentist use if you are undertaking treatment for porcelain veneers, crowns, or dental implants?

- What does the dentist charge for treatments?

Now, if you have gotten as far as a consultation, there are a few more questions you should consider before committing to treatment.

Did the dentist explain all his or her treatment options as well as the advantages and disadvantages of the choice of treatment?

Did he or she explain the treatment process, and did he or she say how long the new porcelain veneers, crowns, or tooth whitening would last? [4]

4   My thanks to my colleague Dr. Tom Orent, www.GoldAutoPilot.com, from whom the above "14 Questions You Must Ask" is adapted (based in part upon his "7 Critical Questions You Must Ask").

7

WHERE TO LOOK WHEN SEARCHING FOR YOUR PERFECT DENTIST

Many of the recommendations to follow will utilise cosmetic dentistry as an illustration. Please note, my recommendations are relevant to all areas of dentistry, whether you are looking for a gum specialist, a dentist who replaces missing teeth with implants, or a cosmetic dentist.

There are a number of sources offering recommendations and advice, the most common being:

- Recommendations from friends and family
- General advertising
- The Internet
- Dentists featured on TV, magazines, and newspaper articles

Recommendations from Friends and Family

Most people will know of a general dentist who can provide fillings, crowns, and remove teeth if required; however, if the consumer has not personally experienced cosmetic dentistry before, it can be difficult to recommend a quality cosmetic dentist.

When it comes to trusting a dentist with your smile, it is only natural to want a dentist who has extensive experience in cosmetic dentistry. After all, it is your smile, and you want to look and feel great afterward, not end up with a terrible smile that makes you feel worse or teeth you can't eat or talk with.

You may have already realised when researching this subject that nearly all dentists offer cosmetic dentistry. What you may not know is that there are approximately thirty-six thousand registered dentists in the UK. Out of these thirty-six thousand dentists, less than one thousand (less than 3 percent of registered dentists) are active members of the British Academy of Cosmetic Dentistry (BACD) and British Academy of Aesthetic Dentistry (BAAD). These are the two leading organisations in the UK actively educating dentists in the art and science of cosmetic dentistry.

When looking for a cosmetic dentist or any other type of dental treatment, most people will start by asking friends and family. This is a good place to start, especially if you know someone who has experienced the type of treatment you are looking for.

It is important to ask that person the right questions about his or her dentist, the most important being:

- What types of treatment does the dentist offer?
- How experienced is the dentist in the treatment you are seeking?
- Did the dentist explain all his or her treatment options as well as the advantages and disadvantages of their treatment of choice?
- Did the dentist explain the treatment process, and did he or she say how long the new porcelain veneers, crowns, dental implants, or tooth whitening would last?
- Does the dentist offer any form of consumer protection, and if so, for how long and what are the terms and conditions?

One common mistake is to solely judge one's recommendation on whether the dentist is nice, or whether he or she causes no pain. Sure, if a friend or family member likes his or her dentist, then you probably will too, and we all want to be treated by a kind, gentle person. However, this is not a good enough reason to act on that recommendation alone. The dentist may have no experience in the type of treatment you are looking for.

You may choose a particular dentist on a recommendation by a friend or family member for cosmetic or dental implant treatment. The recommendation may be based on the fact that he or she is the nicest dentist in the world, but if he or she only treats two or three cosmetic cases per year, are you going to receive the best- looking smile possible?

If you are reading this book, then you have probably already asked friends and family but have found their recommendations unsuitable. They may not know any suitable dentists, or recommend their own general dentist who has little experience with cosmetic treatments or dental implants. So where do you look next?

General Advertising

Considering a dentist you have seen in an advertisement is one way to choose your perfect dentist. General advertising takes many forms of media, from advertisements in newspapers and magazines, to radio and television. If you happen to be looking for dental treatment, then it may be worth taking note of a particular advertisement.

There is nothing wrong with choosing a dentist based on an advertisement you have seen as long as you take the time to research the choice you have made. Jumping straight in to a decision based solely on the information in an advertisement is like playing Russian roulette—on one hand, you may be lucky and find exactly what you are looking for, but on the other hand, you may find you have made a terrible mistake.

Advertisements will often list a dentist's name, contact information, and Web address. Use such advertisements as a starting point by taking note of the information available, then search online, check the GDC register, and follow the advice in this book before making a final decision.

The Internet

The Internet offers an extensive source of information, *but beware!* How many times have you visited a Web site to find out later that things are not all what they seem? The Web is full of fraudulent and immoral people making bold claims. Any self-respecting, ethical dentist would never do such a thing—or would he?

The General Dental Council (GDC) has the power to remove any dentist from the dental register (take away his licence to practice) if found to be publishing fraudulent claims or information. However, at present any dentist can state he offers cosmetic or dental implant treatment regardless of his experience, as there is no recognised specialty in these particular fields.

Offering tooth whitening is cosmetic dentistry, but so is a complete smile makeover with porcelain laminate veneers. Just because a dentist possesses experience in tooth whitening does not mean he or she possesses experience with complete smile makeovers. You must therefore dig deeper to find out exactly what his or her level of experience and expertise is.

The Internet is a valuable source of information. If you keep consumer warnings in mind, the Internet allows you to compare many dentists offering similar services and find out exactly what a treatment involves.

If you search Google under the term "cosmetic dentist," or any other type of dentist you are looking for, chances are you will uncover a list of hosting sites. An example of a hosting site is *www. CosmeticDentistryGuide.co.uk.* This site lists the names and contact details of dentists offering cosmetic dentistry in the UK.

This type of hosting site is a great source to look through as a perspective patient, as it enables an easy comparison of services from different dentists while offering technical information about the types of procedures available. I personally pay to list my own dental practice, The Clifton Dental Studio at *www.CliftonSmiles.com,* on this site as well as a number of other similar sites, as they enable many perspective patients to decide whether I offer the right services for them.

The best way to describe this type of site is as a Yellow Pages of cosmetic dentists, and like the Yellow Pages, a dentist must pay to be listed on it. It is therefore important to note that just because a dentist is listed on this type of site does not automatically make him or her an expert in any particular field. He or she is listed solely on the basis that he or she has paid to be there.

An alternative to this type of hosting site is a site like *www. MyPerfectDentist.com.* This shares some similarities to other sites, but it also differs in a number of unique ways. Among the commonalities, dentists pay to be listed on a general dentist search register. You are then free to search the register until you come across a dentist meeting your requirements. The site offers a comprehensive list of general and specialist dentists offering the full complement of dental services, from cosmetic dentistry, implant dentistry, and child dentistry to specialist periodontists, endodontists, and orthodontists, to even bad breath and the treatment of headaches.

What makes this site different is that it also offers a unique "find a dentist" service whereby you register with the site providing contact details and details of the services and types of treatment you are interested in. For an administration fee, a personal introduction between you and a dentist fulfilling your requirements is made.

Dentists recommended by this service are thought of and accepted as experts or specialists in their field of practice by their peers. You can even choose to visit the dentist's dentists—the dentists other dentists go to for treatment when they need fillings, crowns, and implants. Choosing to undertake treatment with dentists recommended by this service ensures you will experience the best possible care available, whether you are looking for dental implants, cosmetic dentistry, or even dentistry for anxious or phobic patients.

In the interest of disclosure and maintaining an unbiased position, as I have attempted to do throughout this book, I wish to declare that I hold a personal and financial interest in *www.MyPefectDentist.com.*

Online Rating or Ranking Sites

A new trend is developing online with the appearance of rating or ranking sites. These sites exist for people to comment and rate their experiences on anything from restaurants to buying a new television to visiting the dentist.

At face value, these sites appear to be a good idea and offer any perspective customer or patient valuable and accurate information. I cannot profess to be an expert on this issue, but in my opinion, they appear to publish biased information toward the negative, or there are too few comments to represent a balanced view. The majority of comments I have noted from American sites appear to be critical from unhappy customers or patients, with very few or no positive comments at all. In time this is a situation that may change. As the popularity of these sites continues to grow (with more and more people posting comments) a more balanced view may emerge. Examples of such sites found on the web using Google are *www.DoctorScorecard.com* and *www.Ratemds.com*. One such site recently established in the UK is *www.IWantGreatCare.org*.

The best advice I can offer at this time is to use these sites with caution and take the information offered at face value. You will be better served by utilising the advice offered in this book to make an informed choice about any perspective dentist rather than taking note of what amounts to unsubstantiated claims and gossip.

> **Please note:** I have no affiliation with any ranking sites. Any sites listed are used for illustration purposes only. Any mention of these sites neither suggests nor implies that information posted on them is inaccurate, misleading, or fraudulent.

Dentists Featured in the General Media

One way to choose a dentist is to seek out those dentists who have been featured as expert guests in magazines, newspapers, television, and radio.

I know many of the dentists who have been featured in magazines, on television, and on the radio. Most offer quality care and service, but this is not a guarantee they all do.

As a dentist, it is possible to buy this kind of media exposure by using a public relations agent. For a fee, a PR agent will introduce a dentist seeking publicity to the journalists responsible for writing articles for magazines like *Vogue* or the producers responsible for television shows like *Ten Years Younger*.

If you have chosen a dentist based on what you have seen and heard in magazines, television, and radio, my advice is to research them further using the recommended questions in this book. That way you can be confident you have made the right decision for you.

8

WHAT YOUR DENTIST
SHOULD DO NEXT

So you have now researched and found a dentist you feel is right for you, and you have asked all the right questions and received the answers you were looking for. What should you now expect from your first visit and consultation?

Depending what type of treatment you are looking to undertake, your new dentist is likely to recommend a comprehensive dental health examination. In fact, it is medical legal requirement that some form of dental health examination be completed by your dentist before proceeding with any treatment.

Even though different treatments require different diagnostic investigations, a comprehensive dental health exam is just that—a thorough examination of all aspects of your dental health. Whether you are aware of a broken filling that you just want to have fixed, or are looking to undertake an elective cosmetic dental procedure, your new dentist should complete a thorough dental health screening to collect as much information as possible regarding the current state of your dental health. Without this type of examination, you may find that diseased teeth, gums, jaw joints, and general health problems go undetected and thus untreated.

Before you accept any advice and treatment from your new dentist, use this examination process to confirm your final decision and choice is a correct one. This examination process will not only allow your new dentist to gather information about you and your dental health, but it will allow you to assess your dentist. A comprehensive examination, which includes some or all of the following tests, is a good indication that your dentist will offer you the best in quality and care.

Some of these tests are considered mandatory—for example, an oral cancer screening—while others are selected when considering a specific treatment like cosmetic dentistry.

Tests that may be included as part of any dentist's comprehensive dental health examination include:

- A clinical examination
- Multiple individual tooth X-rays to provide a complete look at the teeth and area between them
- Moulds of your teeth known as diagnostic or study models. These help a dentist assess the relationship between upper and lower teeth, relationship of the jaws to the skull, tooth position, and any problems relating to the chewing mechanism
- Oral cancer screening
- Registration of your bite to confirm how the upper and lower teeth touch
- Jaw joints health evaluation
- Decay evaluation
- Periodontal (gum) disease and infection analysis
- Examination of the tissues and muscles of the head, face, and neck
- Headache evaluation
- Evaluation photographs of the entire mouth and smile
- Assessment of clenching and grinding habits
- Smile design analysis
- Tooth colour, size, and shape evaluation
- Evaluation of smile to facial type, complexion, and shape

- Evaluation of dental problems contributing to general overall body health
- Bad breath assessment

Depending on the types of treatment you decide to undertake, you may find your new dentist will ask for additional tests to those already listed. For example, if undertaking dental implant treatment, you may require a CT scan (a highly accurate 3D X-ray) to help plan treatment or a dental bacteria test if suffering from gum disease.

To Summarise:

Take this opportunity to assess your new dentist in the early stages of consultation. This is a vital part of the treatment process and thus a good indication of the quality and care you will receive through your entire treatment journey.

9

DENTAL TOURISM—WHAT YOU MUST KNOW BEFORE CONSIDERING TREATMENT ABROAD

The idea of saving hundreds or even thousands of pounds combining a trip to the dentist while enjoying a holiday abroad can sound very appealing. However, there are a number of vital issues you must consider before jetting off for that "bargain" replacement filling, dental implant, or gleaming new smile.

Issues of greatest concern relate to the quality of care you will receive, the increase risk of complications associated with flying after surgery, the availability and standard of after-care on your return to the UK, what happens if things do go wrong, and are you able to make a complaint or seek recourse if the worst should happen.

Many patients seeking care abroad have found it to be a satisfactory experience, but some have found themselves returning to the UK with considerable problems from complications or inappropriate care. To make matters worse, they have then required additional treatment at considerable cost to fix their problems back in the UK.

As a dentist, my advice would always be to stay at home for treatment.

However, if you are determined to undertake treatment abroad you should always choose a country where training and standards of care are accepted as equivalent to that offered in the UK. You should then insist that the following questions are answered to your complete satisfaction before proceeding with treatment.

Nine Questions You Must Ask before Traveling Abroad for Treatment

1. **Who will be completing your treatment, and what qualifications does he or she hold?**

   The first thing you should do is research the dentist you are considering treatment with. It is important to establish what qualifications he holds and check whether these are recognised by the GDC or equivalent to those held by dentists in the UK.

2. **Is the dentist regulated by a professional body, and if so, is compulsory registration required?**

   In the UK all dentists are regulated by and must be registered with the General Dental Council (GDC). The GDC is responsible for setting and upholding the standards to which all UK dentists must practice. As a dental tourist, it is critical that you undertake treatment with a dentist who is regulated to the appropriate standards of care.

   You can find out about health regulators and professional bodies in other countries by visiting *www.HealthRegulation. org*. If a health regulator does exist, you should be able find the professional body responsible for dental health care and the standards of care they enforce.

3. **Will you be able to communicate in English, and if not, will an interpreter be supplied?**

   Good communication is a necessity if you are to understand and be fully informed about proposed treatments (whether in the UK or abroad). If your first and only language is English, then it is imperative that the dentist and his or her team speak English, or that an interpreter be supplied.

4. **What are the success rates of treatment and the likelihood of complications?**

    You may find that quality of care, techniques, and the materials employed by some dentists abroad do not reach the same clinical standards to those in UK. It is therefore important to always confirm the success rates and likelihood of complications before proceeding with treatment, as you may find they fall short of that normally expected by a dentist at home.

5. **What level of aftercare service is available, and is care available on return to the UK?**

    Depending on the type of procedure you undertake, quality aftercare may be a necessity. If so, will you need to fly back abroad for aftercare, or is care available within the UK? If abroad, will you need to pay for additional flights and accommodation, or is this included within your original quotation? You should check this carefully, as you may find the original savings are not as great as first thought.

6. **What happens if complications do arise? Who is responsible for the cost of flights, travel, and hotel arrangements, including any remedial work required in the UK upon your return?**

    If a complication arises following treatment abroad, it is important that you will be looked after. As with aftercare, it is important to check whom you should seek help from if an acute emergency arises. If additional care is required, you should take great care to confirm who is responsible for your welfare once back in the UK and the costs involved. If the worst should happen, you do not want to find yourself in a situation where you cannot find a dentist to help, or in a position where you cannot afford the additional treatment required to correct a problem.

7. **Does the dentist possess indemnity cover or malpractice insurance to protect patients?**

Assuming you are entitled to recourse (depending on the country you undertake treatment in), check if the dentist is indemnified or if he or she possess malpractice insurance. Both indemnity and malpractice insurance provide you, the patient, with protection if the worst should happen. However, there are a few key differences between indemnity cover and insurance that you should be aware of.

Indemnity cover is provided by non-profit mutual associations owned by its members, whereas profit-focused commercial organisations, such as insurance companies, are answerable to the financial interests of shareholders. Anyone who has made an insurance claim will be aware that commercial insurance companies assess each claim against the carefully worded clauses of each policy. The wording of any insurance policy intentionally defines and thereby limits cover. As such, you may find your level of protection is strictly limited.

In comparison, indemnity through a mutual association allows greater flexibility, enabling assistance (and compensation) to be given in circumstances that would not be covered within a contractual insurance situation. The largest organisation offering indemnity cover in the UK (Dental Protection) also offers an added benefit to all member dentists and therefore patients. When a dentist ceases to practice (e.g., retirement), he or she is no longer obliged to pay additional premiums to cover all patients treated under his or her care (no matter how long he or she has been retired). In comparison, a dentist who was covered by insurance and is now retired must continue to either pay a premium for continued cover or purchase an alternative policy to protect his or her patients. If the dentist fails to do this (and there is no obligation to do so), you the patient are no longer protected.

This last point is important to note: You may find that short-term savings are to be had by undertaking treatment abroad, but in the longer term, you may not be protected and therefore subject to significant costs if something were to go wrong.

Because of these benefits, around 70 percent of all dentists in the UK possess indemnity with the Dental Protection (a mutual society) in preference to insurance cover.

Although aimed primarily at dentists, additional information regarding indemnity versus insurance can be found under the heading Insurance Vs. Indemnity at *www.DentalProtection.org*.

It is a statutory registration requirement with the General Dental Council (GDC) that all dentists practicing in the UK must possess indemnity or malpractice insurance.

> **Please note;** other countries hold their own statutory requirements which do not always require a dentist to possess indemnity or malpractice insurance in the interests of patient protection.

8. **Does the dentist possess a robust complaints procedure, and if so, is a copy available?**

    Turn to section six to see the robust complaints procedures available to all patients treated by dentists within the UK. If undertaking treatment abroad, you should confirm the existence of a complaints procedure and whether it offers you the ability to voice your concerns and then have those concerns acted upon.

9. **Who do you go to for advice following treatment?**

    Again, it is important to confirm that a point of contact is available should you need advice following treatment.

To Summarise:

*   Who will be completing your treatment, and what qualifications does he or she hold?

*   Is the dentist regulated by a professional body, and if so, is compulsory registration required?

- Will you be able to communicate in English, and if not, will an interpreter be supplied?

- What are the success rates of treatment and the likelihood of complications?

- What level of aftercare service is available, and is care available on return to the UK?

- What happens if complications do arise? Who is responsible for the cost of flights, travel, and hotel arrangements, including any remedial work required in the UK upon your return?

- Does the dentist possess indemnity cover or malpractice insurance to protect patients?

- Does the dentist possess a robust complaints procedure, and if so, is a copy available?

- Who do you go to for advice following treatment?

In addition to these questions, do not forget to follow the advice already outlined in this book.

Further information is available through the General Dental Council (GDC) at *www.gdc-uk.org*.

PART THREE

THE NHS, PRIVATE DENTAL CARE, AND DENTAL HEALTH INSURANCE

10

THE NATIONAL HEALTH SERVICE (NHS)

Before I comment on the National Health Service (NHS), in particular NHS dentistry, I would like to make it clear that I support the NHS and feel it offers an invaluable service.

Virtually all health professionals, whether they are nurses, doctors, or dentists and the many support staff you never see or hear about, work under compromised conditions every day. They find themselves overworked, understaffed, and undervalued by the powers that be, but they consistently offer their time in the best interests of their patients above that of their own.

The ideology behind the NHS is free access to quality medical and dental health care regardless of wealth and status. While this is a worthy cause, it is an impossible dream. No matter how politicians and governments try to dress it up, we are all aware of the desperate situation in which the NHS currently finds itself. Not a week passes by where we do not hear about failings within the NHS. This is a situation that may worsen still when the significant cutbacks in public spending start to bite following the recent economic turmoil.

In my opinion, the most significant factors that prevent the dream from becoming a reality are the costs of running a "free" at-point-of-access high quality service to all, and the willingness of individuals to take responsibility for their own health and well-being.

NHS medicine and dentistry will always be a bottomless pit of money where demand will continue to outstrip supply. We as a population are growing while also living longer, thus placing an ever-increasing demand on resources. As medicine and dentistry advance, the costs of new technologies become prohibitive, thus leading to a rationing of service.

Even countries like France, regarded as having one of the best health services in the world, now finds itself considering cutbacks, no longer able to afford and maintain the standard of care it currently offers.

So, with only finite resources, do you spend the money on life-saving treatments or help an individual to chew or feel better when smiling in the mirror? I cannot offer you any answers, as it can be argued that an individual's psychological state of mind is fundamental to his or her general health and well-being. Ultimately, though, dentistry will always be relegated to a low priority service when held alongside life-saving treatments for diseases like cancer and heart disease.

It can also be argued that we as a population take little responsibility for our own health and well-being. Many people's lifestyles and social activities lead to otherwise preventable medical and dental diseases. For example, smoking, excessive alcohol consumption, and obesity are all responsible for many of the illnesses the NHS deals with on a daily basis.

Hundreds of millions of pounds of confectionary are purchased each year. Everyone knows that sweets and sugar are bad for your teeth; so why do we see so much dental disease? Another hard-to-believe example is the number of toothbrushes sold within the UK each year. Most recent figures indicate that we buy around 117 million toothbrushes per year, on average just two toothbrushes per person. Considering that many people change their toothbrush every eight to twelve weeks as advised by their dentist, one can only conclude that literally millions of people neither own nor use a toothbrush.[5]

NHS Dental Care

With around 60 percent of all dental procedures completed annually under the NHS, there is an obvious demand for NHS dental care within the UK. However, the provision of NHS dentistry in the UK has been a contentious issue for over twenty years, with

---

5   Data supplied Courtesy Oral-B and IRI Major Multiples. Data to December 26, 2009.

patients, dentists, and politicians alike questioning the value and quality of service.

Much of this discontent was initiated in the late 1980s and early 1990s, when the then-conservative government forced significant changes upon the dental profession. This limited the ability of dentists to offer the very best long-term care while increasing direct patient charges, resulting in a significant number of dentists leaving the NHS for private dental care.

Until recently, the failings of successive governments to invest in dentistry had resulted in a situation where not only was the availability of NHS dental care limited in many areas of the country, but quality of available care was compromised due to the continual under-funding of the service.

In an attempt to remedy this situation, the Labour government introduced a new dental contract in April 2006 to England and Wales, promising to increase both funding and access to NHS dentistry. Scotland and Northern Ireland have continued with their own arrangements.

Prior to April 2006, NHS dentists were paid for each treatment they completed. You may be surprised to know that you as a patient paid 80 percent of the cost of any treatment you undertook during this period, while the government paid just 20 percent of the total treatment charge.

Only when treatment costs rose above a set fee of around £370 did the government pay the majority of the cost. So, if you needed large numbers of teeth treated, you benefited; if not, you paid virtually the entire fee, believing your dentist was receiving large subsidies from the NHS. This system possessed many drawbacks, one of which was to place the dentist in a situation where all he could offer was reactive treatment (i.e., treat active problems rather than providing preventive care, treatments to secure good dental health and prevent long-term disease).

Dentists are now paid via a target-driven system, a fixed annual payment in return for fixed number of treatments per year. Each treatment is classified in to one of three levels, to which a different patient charge is attached. Interestingly, this new system was imposed upon the profession without any prior testing and has thus proven to possess its own set of problems, while systems that were extensively tested prior to April 2006 and did appear to show improvement in care quality were rejected.

Given the time lapse between writing and publishing, it is impossible for a book to be perfectly current. At the time of writing, government data indicates that access to NHS dentistry is struggling to reach pre-2006 levels, while an increase in "simple" treatments has increased at the expense of "complex" treatments. The data suggests that instead of saving more teeth, an increased number of teeth are actually being removed.

There is still disagreement between the government and dental profession over the true meaning of these figures, but as yet evidence supporting a significant improvement is inconclusive.

On a more positive note, the government appears to be committed to further improvement of NHS dentistry, commissioning new pilot schemes designed to improve both the quality and care of dental services.

Choosing the Perfect NHS Dentist

Due to my interests in cosmetic and implant dentistry, much of this book is orientated to private dental care. However, you may find that a number of my recommendations are suitable for choosing an NHS dentist—for example, checking to see if the dentist is registered with the GDC, searching online for an NHS dentist, confirming how many years he or she has been performing the procedure you are interested in, or seeking testimonials from other grateful patients.

You may find your choices limited by the availability of NHS dental care. Access and therefore choice in NHS care varies widely in different regions of the country. If good access is available within a region, then the option to choose your perfect dentist may be possible. If access is very limited or nonexistent, then you have little choice other than to choose the only available NHS dentist or seek alternative private arrangements.

11

FIVE REASONS TO CONSIDER PRIVATE DENTISTRY

There are many benefits for choosing private dentistry, especially if you use this book as intended to seek out the right dentist for you. The most significant benefits are the availability of a dentist's time and the range of treatments offered.

Understandably, due to financial limitations, NHS dentistry cannot offer cosmetic or dental implant-related treatments (except in a very small number of unique cases within a hospital environment (e.g., adolescents with hereditary missing adult teeth). When considering cosmetic dentistry or tooth replacement with dental implants, you will find these services available through private dental care only.

As a private dentist, I do not see more than ten patients per day. This allows me to dedicate the time I need to provide the high quality service demanded by my patients. But what does that statement really mean?

It means:

- I have the time to ask you as a patient what you are looking for, what problems you have, and how you would like to fix them. I have time to consider your thoughts, feelings, and long-term goals.

- I have the time to explain all treatment options available to you. There is normally more than one way to treat the same problem. Some options will ultimately be better than others, but it provides you as a patient with the information you need to make an informed choice—all the information you need to make the right decision for you.

- I have the time to complete all treatments to the same high standards I use when treating my wife and family—the same standards I would expect if I was receiving treatment myself.

- I have the time to use techniques that make treatment as pain-free and as comfortable as possible. Nobody likes dental treatment, and offering pain-free treatment takes more time (e.g., if you rush an injection, it hurts; take the time to administer it very slowly and you will feel very little or no pain at all).

- Finally, depending on your choice of treatment, I have the ability to use the best techniques and materials, which ultimately look better, feel better, and often last significantly longer, thus reducing the need for additional long-term treatment.

Let me ask you a question. As a patient, would you rather receive treatment that minimises the chances of further problems, that looks and feels great while lasting as long as possible? Or would you prefer a quick fix that may result in more damage and disease in the long term, resulting in the need for dental treatment more often with a greater chance of toothache and the loss of teeth?

Only you can decide what best meets your requirements, but many of my patients choose the former option. Treating low numbers of patients enables me to offer this level of care, a level of quality demanded by the people seeking my services.

If I have yet to convince you of the value of private care and why you should consider it, then consider this widely quoted business model (used by economists and businesses worldwide) seen in Figure 1.

Fig 1

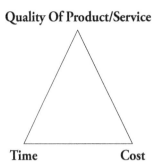

Quality Of Product/Service

Time   **Cost**

This triangle describes the following features of quality of service or product versus time versus cost. In an ideal world, when buying any product or service, whether you are in a restaurant, purchasing a new pair of shoes, or undertaking dental treatment, you would want the very best possible service and quality of product in the shortest period of time at the lowest possible cost.

Unfortunately, the reality is such that you can only ever possess two of these features together at any one time. Therefore, taking dentistry as an example, it is possible to buy a crown or filling quickly and at low cost, but to achieve this, it will likely be of low quality. In this instance, low quality may mean it fits poorly, wears out quickly, or looks unsightly. (As such, there is a higher risk of further tooth decay, toothache, and potential loss of a tooth.)

Alternatively, you may decide you want the very best crown or filling because you value your dental health. It is still possible to have this in a relatively short time frame, but you must pay a much higher cost if you want it to look great while fitting perfectly, thus lasting as long as possible.

12

THE COST OF A HEALTHY MOUTH AND SMILE

In the UK, there is a general perception that private dental care is an expensive option when considering treatment.

Admittedly, some cosmetic dental treatments, like a smile makeover, can be costly, perhaps even of equal cost to a new car, but I will always support the statement that quality private dental care offers good value for money. Higher cost does not mean poor value for money; it is quite the opposite, in fact. I would argue that low cost normally results in poor value for money, as most products and services produced at low cost can only be of low cost for three reasons: Either the quality of the product is poor or entirely absent, the service is severely lacking or nonexistent, or the time taken for the product or service to be delivered is way beyond that normally considered to be acceptable.

Affordability

The majority of us are in a position to buy what we want. I do not mean we all have the means to buy everything we want all of the time, but most of us can afford some of the things we want some of the time.

Most of us find ourselves in the position where we will sacrifice those things of least importance for those of greatest importance. For example, if we choose to purchase a new television this year, we may find that we can only eat out at restaurants once per month instead of once a week, or if we want something a little costlier like a holiday this year, we may have to go without a new kitchen. If we buy a new car this year, we may have to keep the existing kitchen and go without a holiday. I can go on, but you get the idea.

So, in general terms, most things are an affordable option if you want it and feel it is of real value.

How Valuable Is Your Health?

Private dental care is one of those things that is affordable if you want it and feel it is of real value. So, at what price do you value your smile and general dental health? If you are struggling to come to a decision, let me ask you a question that may help you place a value on your dental health and the quality of dental care you would ideally like to receive.

How much would I have to pay you for you to let me take out one of your healthy front teeth? If I offered you £100 to let me take out one front tooth, would this be acceptable? Or is £1,000 closer to the mark? I bet your reaction is considerably greater than £1,000, and even then you would want a new tooth put back in its place.

Only you can decide the level of care that is right for you. So long as you understand your available options and the compromises you may be asked to make, then there is no right or wrong answer.

Private Dental Fees

I cannot tell you what you should pay for any particular type of private dental treatment, as there will always be a variation in what each dentist charges for the same procedure. Each dentist will set his or her fees at a level that represents his or her skill and experience, the quality of care provided, and the costs of running a private dental practice. The fees you pay will very much depend on the quality of care you wish to receive. So, a good starting point is to decide what that level of care is.

It is important to note that each treatment is bespoke to the individual and not a commodity manufactured at high volume on a production line. It is therefore impossible to truly compare a like for like service based on cost alone. In fact, making a judgment on cost alone is the worst way to make a decision regarding your health, but it may help you to identify a standard of care meeting your requirements.

The best advice I can offer when searching for your perfect dentist is to use the information in this book to compare services, quality of care offered, experience of the dentist, and results of previous patients, rather than price. This will not only provide you with a feel for what you should be looking for, but will also provide you with a better idea of the quality you are likely to receive for the budget you have in mind.

To Summarise:
- When searching for your perfect dentist, always compare the following, rather than costs alone:
- Available treatments/services
- Quality of care offered
- Experience of the dentist
- Results of previous patients

13

DENTAL HEALTH INSURANCE

Many prospective patients ask me about dental health insurance. The most common questions are: is it worth having, and what treatment will it cover?

There are generally two types of dental insurance. The first is a conventional dental health policy offered by reputable health insurance providers such as Simplyhealth, AXA, and Aviva. The second type is insurance linked to a monthly payment plan through your dentist. A well-known example of this is Denplan.

What Are the Differences and Benefits of the Two?

Conventional Insurance

A conventional dental insurance policy must be organised and purchased by you, either through an insurance broker or directly from the insurance company. You will pay a fixed annual premium, which will normally cover a percentage of any treatment costs incurred or pay a fixed amount toward a particular type of treatment.

For example, if a back tooth were to need a crown or filling, your insurance may pay 50 percent of the total cost of treatment up to a maximum value of £500. Alternatively, they may pay a fixed amount toward the cost of each itemised treatment. They may pay a fixed fee of £250 toward the cost of a crown, whether the crown costs £500 or £1,000. All dental insurance provided in this way will cap the total amount payable in any given year (normally £500 to £2,000 per annum).

The advantage of conventional dental insurance is that you are the policyholder. This means you can claim for treatment provided by any dentist (you do not need to be a member of one particular dental practice). For example, if you see your regular dentist but require specialised treatment that he or she does not provide, he or she can refer you to a registered specialist for treatment that can still be claimed against your insurance policy.

Another advantage is that in most cases almost anyone can purchase this type of insurance without a dental health examination. Insurance coverage is not normally subject to the existing condition of your teeth.

The disadvantages of conventional dental insurance are similar to that of any insurance policy. Insurance companies exist to make money. They understand that quality dental care can be costly and will often place severe restrictions on what they will pay for. If you possess healthy teeth, you may find you will never benefit from the premiums you pay.

An important point to note is that conventional insurance policies do not offer immediate cover and are unlikely to pay for any existing condition under active treatment. In most cases, you will not be able to claim for any treatment for a minimum of three months from the time you purchase the policy. You will likely find that there are also age restrictions, with coverage only available up to seventy years of age.

The one situation in which most insurance providers are often very generous is accidental injury. The chances of you accidentally injuring your teeth as an adult have been reported as high as 10 percent. This means one in every ten adults will accidentally damage their smile at some point in life from such activities as falling off of a bike, a sports injury, a car accident, or even physical assault. For children this statistic is even higher, with around one in every three children damaging their teeth.[6]

---

6 Bastone, Elisa B., Terry J. Freer, and John R. McNamara. "Epidemology of Dental Trauma: A Review of the Literature." *Australian Dental Journal.* 2000, 45 (1): 2–9.

Insurance Linked to a Monthly Payment Plan Directly through a Dentist

Denplan is just one example of a number of monthly payment plans offered to patients by many dentists throughout the UK. Normal requirements for this type of policy insist that you be a regular attending patient of a practice or individual dentist. The benefits of this type of policy are that regular dental health assessments and hygiene sessions are inclusive within the monthly premiums you pay. They will normally cover the complete costs of most treatments without annual limits (with additional fees for crowns and other laboratory work—depending on membership level). Coverage will normally start immediately, there is no age limit and again, and accidental injury insurance is often included and generous. (Please check the specifics of any payment plan to confirm this.)

The disadvantage to this type of insurance/payment plan is that it is underwritten by your dentist, and as such it will only cover treatments provided by your dentist. If you wish to visit a new dental practice or undertake treatment with a registered dental specialist, you will not be covered. One exception to this is treatment relating to accidental injury. Under these circumstances, you may be covered for treatment with another dentist or registered dental specialist if your own dentist cannot provide the care you require. (Again, please check the specifics of any policy/plan to confirm this.)

Another disadvantage to this type of insurance/payment plan is the more treatment your dentist completes, the less money he will make from your monthly premium. This type of plan is therefore open to abuse and can result in supervised neglect. The term "supervised neglect" describes a situation where a dentist diagnoses disease but chooses to either treat it in a very limited fashion (a short-term patch-up) or ignore it altogether if it causes no obvious pain or immediate problems.

This type of plan, therefore, requires your dentist to uphold the highest ethical standards. To be fair, dentists sincerely care about the patients they treat; however, the General Dental Council (GDC) has found it necessary to remove dentists from the dental register (take away their license to practice) due to long-term supervised neglect.

The best advice I can offer you is similar to that for any insurance. Carefully consider your risks against the benefits you will receive for the premium you will pay. You may find you will be better served without insurance, saving the money you would pay toward the premium in the longer term, as it is likely you will be no worse off. If treatment is then required, you have the option to choose the treatment that is in your best interest, rather than what is in the best interest of the insurance company or dentist.

One additional common question I hear is: will my insurance pay for cosmetic dentistry? As cosmetic dentistry is an elective procedure not necessary for dental health, no insurance policy will pay for cosmetic treatments. They will only cover health-related problems. You are also likely to find that most policies will not cover treatments involving dental implants, although some may offer restricted cover at an increased premium.

Maintenance Plans

An alternative approach I advocate in preference to any insurance is a monthly maintenance payment plan. This type of plan is provided through your dentist, enabling you to spread the cost of routine dental health assessments and hygiene sessions. It is designed to provide preventive treatment only, treatments to reduce the chance of you needing active dental treatment in the future. You then pay for active treatment like fillings and crowns if and when required (normally at a preferential rate if you are a member of this type of plan). These plans may be branded (e.g., Denplan essentials) or offered as an in-house product of a practice.

Please note: I have no affiliation with any insurance company or insurance/payment plan provider. Due to the inevitable time lapse between drafting and publishing of a book, some of my comments relating to dental insurance may no longer be applicable. As such, the information provided in this chapter is for illustration purposes only. The specific details and benefits of any policy should be confirmed on an individual basis before and at the time of purchase.

PART FOUR

DEFEATING FEAR
OF THE DENTIST

14

FIVE WAYS TO DEFEAT FEAR OF THE DENTIST

Don't Let Fear of the Dentist Prevent You from Having the Perfect Healthy Smile

Are you petrified of the dentist? Do you feel sick, experience palpitations, or get sweaty palms at just the thought of dental treatment? Have you ever missed a dental appointment because of uncontrollable fear? Or do you attend appointments but feel anxious the entire time? If so, you are not alone.

If you class yourself as a dental phobic and you have summoned the courage to read this book, then congratulations. If you are not, but know someone who is, keep reading. You may just find that the following information will help you transform the life of a friend or family member.

Whether you are interested in cosmetic treatments or routine dental care, it matters not. Millions of people from all walks of life suffer with fear of the dentist on a daily basis, to a point that some cannot control the way they feel or behave, whether visiting a dentist or just thinking about it.

The reasons for this can be complex, but many of these fears are a result of a previous dental experiences found to be unpleasant in some way. This is known as a conditioned fear, often learned during childhood. Subsequently those feelings associated with that experience can develop to the point at which a phobia develops.

A phobia can be described as an anxiety disorder characterised by extreme and irrational fear of simple things or social situations. A phobia affects people's lives quite differently than fear or general anxiety. Fear of the dentist, for example, will not stop someone from walking past a dental practice or looking at a dental advertisement in a magazine, or even undertaking treatment. Fears can be overcome with increased familiarity of a situation, whereas a phobia cannot. Phobias result in such intense anxiety or panic attacks that the sufferer must avoid the situation altogether. For example, true dental phobics can experience these symptoms at just the thought of dental treatment, looking at a dental advertisement, or walking past a dental practice. It will literally control their behaviour, to the point that they would rather suffer agonising toothache than seek help from a dentist.

As a dentist, I completely relate to this, not through a fear of dental treatment, but like many, I possess a fear of flying. As with many fears, I experience similar physical symptoms and feelings when flying to those of the anxious dental patient. I understand these feelings are totally irrational, but this has little influence over the way I feel. These feelings are beyond control of rational thought.

So, how do you defeat fear of the dentist? How can you overcome the anxiety many people feel when visiting the dentist or the irrational fear experienced by the dental phobic?

Whether used in isolation or as combined therapy, the following five techniques will help virtually anyone overcome their fear of dental treatment, and they consist of:

- Distraction techniques
- Desensitisation therapy
- Hypnotherapy
- Cognitive behavioural therapy
- Use of medication and dental sedation

15

DISTRACTION TECHNIQUES

Distraction techniques work well for those patients experiencing mild levels of anxiety—the vast majority of people.

Dentists deal with anxious or fearful patients every day. To provide the most comfortable experience possible, many dentists will employ a number of techniques designed to distract patients from their physical surroundings. The aim, to reduce a patient's anxiety and increase his or her comfort by distracting his or her attention from the here and now to stimulate other thoughts and feelings not associated with dental care.

This can be achieved in a number of ways, the most common relating to our senses of sound, smell, and vision. For example, some dentists will use calming music to set a relaxing tone, scented candles or oils to mask surgical smells, while decoration, lighting, and TV/video images are used to redirect a patient's attention.

If I am honest, I don't know of anyone who doesn't experience some level of anxiety when visiting the dentist for treatment, even some dentists themselves! So the use of simple distraction techniques can help everyone to feel that little more relaxed in an otherwise uncomfortable situation.

16

DESENSITISATION THERAPY

Desensitisation techniques work well for those who experience mild to moderate anxiety.

Many of our anxieties develop through a learned association between a particular situation and an object or stimulus. For example, we learn from a young age that an injection is associated with pain. We then associate other stimulus, like the smell of disinfectant used by the dentist with the painful injection, then the sound of the dental drill and the smell of disinfectant with the painful injection, and so on.

Desensitisation therapy aims to restore a patient's confidence and trust in the dentist and dental treatment by teaching or reinforcing a new positive experience while breaking the association between a particular stimulus and a past negative experience. For example, if a patient undertakes a number of treatments requiring dental anaesthetic and the patient feels no pain from each injection, the patient will not only start to trust the dentist resulting in less anxiety, but the link between the painful injection and visit to the dentist is softened or even broken. The patient is desensitised to the previous negative experience.

It is possible to reduce or eliminate many different anxieties in this way, but to do so demands commitment and patience from both dentist and patient.

These techniques may be used independently or in conjunction with hypnotherapy and CBT for those who experience a greater level of anxiety.

.

17

HYPNOTHERAPY

Hypnotherapy is no longer thought of as wacky mind control by science but as a proven technique for the treatment of a variety of medical and psychological problems. As such, hypnotherapy can be used to great effect in the treatment of dental anxieties or phobias.

Hypnosis works by altering our state of consciousness in such a way that the conscious mind, where intellectual thoughts take place, can be bypassed. This reduces analytical evaluation, allowing access to the behavioural templates stored within the subconscious mind. This is normally achieved through a process of focused concentration or guided imagery. It is a natural state, and most people will report it to be a pleasant experience. The subconscious mind is home to our more primitive thought processes, instincts (those instincts designed to protect us), and patterns of behaviour, and as such, it is the subconscious mind that stores our deep-seated fears and anxieties. Hypnosis allows access to the subconscious mind, which can then, through therapy, be receptive to new ideas and suggestions. Hypnotherapy (therapy through hypnosis) takes advantage of the subconscious mind's susceptibility to suggestion to induce beneficial changes, thus influencing the conscious mind.

For example, a highly anxious/phobic patient can make a determined conscious effort to overcome his or her fear of the dentist, but will often fail to succeed because his or her subconscious mind retains a deep-seated fear. Success is possible once a patient has been taught to manage his or her anxiety, making it possible for the subconscious mind to disassociate from the deep-seated fear response, essentially re-programming the subconscious mind. This enables the replacement of negative thoughts or feelings with positive ones, having a positive influence on the patient's conscious thoughts and behaviors.

Hypnotherapy is a very safe method for treating fear and anxiety. Although hypnosis reduces conscious evaluation, you can never be conditioned or persuaded to do something you do not want to do. The patient ultimately retains control. For simplicity, you may think of a hypnotherapist's role as that of a guide, a facilitator who is trained to help you achieve a hypnotic state of mind, then help you to take control of your own thoughts and feelings at both a conscious and subconscious level.

Limitations of Hypnotherapy

Successful treatment of a condition with hypnotherapy is dependent on an individual's intent to make change alongside his or her susceptibility to suggestion. According to the British Society of Clinical Hypnosis, 85 percent of people will respond to some level of hypnotherapy. This percentage shows that even though hypnotherapy may not be for everyone, a high number of the population will gain some improvement. If you are tired of being controlled by your anxiety and fears, you have nothing to lose by trying hypnotherapy.

Relatively few dentists offer treatment under hypnosis, but that shouldn't be a barrier to hypnotherapy. As all registered hypnotherapists possess the necessary skills to help, there is no reason to stop you visiting one independently.

The British Society of Clinical Hypnosis offers a database of registered hypnotherapists throughout the UK. This list is available online at *www.bsch.org.uk*. Alternatively, you may contact them directly by calling 01262 403103.

My thanks to Stephanie Burton, Clinical Hypnotherapist EDH DHP MNCH (Reg.), of Clifton Hypnotherapy, www.cliftonhypnotherapy.co.uk, for her support and advice with this subject.

18

COGNITIVE BEHAVIORAL THERAPY (CBT)

CBT (a form of psychotherapy) is a very effective treatment for those who experience high levels of anxiety and even phobias.

CBT works by helping you to discover how your thoughts affect the way you feel and subsequently how your feelings affect your behaviour. If you can think about yourself, surroundings, and other people differently, you can affect the way you feel and thus modify your behavior.

Deep-seated dental fear and anxiety may be directly associated with a previous traumatic dental experience but may also result from a past experience completely unrelated to dental care. Whatever the cause, CBT can help you to understand the reasons for your anxieties and provide you with the tools necessary to overcome them.

As a dental phobic, you may not have realised that much of the fear and anxiety you experience when undertaking dental treatment has more to do with fear of the physical symptoms of a panic attack—the fear of palpitations, nausea, hyperventilation, and loss of complete control—rather than fear of treatment itself.

What Does CBT Involve?

CBT can be undertaken with a therapist on an individual basis, within a group or even as a self-help treatment from a book or online.

Individual therapy with a qualified therapist will normally involve five to twenty weekly or fortnightly sessions (each session lasting thirty to sixty minutes). The first few sessions will help you and the therapist decide whether you will benefit from CBT and that you feel comfortable with the experience. Together you will look at your thoughts, feelings, and behaviours to work out if they are unrealistic or unhelpful and how they affect each other and you. Following this, your therapist will help you to work out how to change unhelpful thoughts and behaviors for your long-term benefit.

Fear Fighter is an online program approved by the NHS for the treatment of anxieties and phobias if you prefer the idea of "self-help." For further information, please visit *www.FearFighter.com.*

Limitations of CBT

There are some limitations with CBT.

- Treatment is not a quick fix, as CBT can take many months to complete.

- CBT requires a personal commitment and effort from the individual, and as such, the CBT therapist is there to advise and encourage you only (he or she cannot do it for you).

- Finally, CBT requires you to confront your anxieties, which may make you feel worse in the short term before things get better.

You can find out more about CBT and search for a therapist through the British Association for Behavioural and Cognitive Psychotherapies at *www.babcp.com.* Further information is also available from Royal College of Psychiatrists at *www.rcpsych.ac.uk* .

19

USE OF MEDICATION AND DENTAL SEDATION

The use of medication to control dental fear and anxiety is not new, but we as dentists appear to have been slow to promote its benefits and make it widely available to our patients.

For many patients, the use of medication to reduce or eliminate their fears and anxieties is still the treatment of choice, as it reduces reliance on the patient's own abilities to control his or her symptoms. However, there are still many anxious and even phobic patients who do not realise that a range of medications and techniques are available to help, which include:

- Oral sedation
- Inhalation sedation or relative analgesia—Nitrous Oxide (laughing gas)
- IV sedation (intravenous sedation/conscious sedation)
- General anesthetic (GA)

Oral Sedation

Oral sedation can be a very effective way of reducing anxiety. It is most suited to those with mild to moderate anxiety (those patients who force themselves to visit the dentist but feel anxious and uncomfortable the entire time).

This technique involves the patient swallowing a drug, normally thirty to sixty minutes before the start of dental treatment, to induce a relaxed state. As a patient, you are conscious and still aware of what is going on around you but feel more relaxed and better able to cope. For many the sensation is like that of being a little tipsy following a good bottle of wine, but without the hangover!

The most commonly used drugs are Diazepam (Valium) and Midazolam. Both belong to a group of drugs known as Benzodiazepines. Diazepam is administered in tablet form, while Midazolam is a liquid solution often administered in fruit juice. The dose of each drug is adjusted to take into account both the size/weight and level of anxiety of the patient. Both drugs produce a number of positive effects and are very safe. As well as reducing anxiety, they also act as a muscle relaxant and can also suppress an overactive gag reflex, both helpful when undertaking dental treatment.

The benefit of this type of sedation is that it can be administered very easily and safely by dentists in general practice. As it is taken orally, it is also very comfortable for the individual patient.

Limitations are few but can be significant.

- The time taken for the drug to take effect varies from person to person (as it is absorbed through the stomach). This means the full effect may not be achieved in time for treatment

- It is difficult to judge the exact dosage required to achieve the best results, and the dosage cannot be adjusted during treatment.

- There is also a limit to the dosage than can be prescribed safely, so some patients may require a higher dose of drug than this technique allows.

- It should not be used for children due to unpredictable results (it can actually increase their emotional responses—make them more upset).

- You can experience a drug hangover. The drug does not make you feel physically ill like alcohol, but it can make you feel a little spaced out for a day or two.

If you feel you need some help to control your anxiety, this can be a great option. One way to experience this technique as an anxious patient is to use it for more simple treatments first (e.g., visiting the hygienist). That way you can see if it works for you before undertaking more complex care.

Just like alcohol, these drugs can affect your judgement and reaction times. Therefore, you should not drive of operate machinery for a minimum of twenty-four hours following treatment.

Inhalation Sedation—Nitrous Oxide (Laughing Gas)

Nitrous Oxide is suitable for mild to moderate/severe anxiety in both adults and children.

This technique involves the administration of Nitrous Oxide gas (which can indeed make you laugh) through a small mask fitted over the nose. Within just a few minutes, you will start to experience a euphoric feeling; you may also feel like you are floating and find that your fingers and toes tingle. As with oral sedation, you are conscious throughout treatment.

The benefits of this type of anxiety control are numerous:

- Nitrous oxide works rapidly, reaching the brain in around twenty seconds, with pain control and euphoria developing in just a few minutes.

- The depth of sedation can be controlled moment to moment; the dose increased or decreased as treatment progresses, offering more control to the dentist and you.

- The effects of the gas wear off rapidly after treatment (within just a few minutes), so you can drive home safely.

- There are no hangover effects as with some drugs, like Diazepam.

- Gag reflex can be reduced

- As nitrous oxide is a pain killer, it can reduce the need for local anaesthetic (e.g., sensitivity during hygiene treatments).

- The technique is extremely safe

There are few limitations, but it is worth mentioning that some people find it does not work sufficiently to help their anxiety. The effects of the gas can also cause nausea and vomiting, while you must be able to breathe sufficiently through your nose. Finally, availability is limited within the UK.

Where possible, this is the treatment of choice for anxious children, as unlike oral sedation, there are no adverse side effects while the results are more predictable.

IV Sedation (Intravenous Sedation/Conscious Sedation)

IV sedation is a very effective and safe way of treating those with moderate to severe anxiety and even phobia. Treatment of anxiety in this way is so effective that it has replaced the use of general anaesthetic in general practice. In fact, it is so effective that virtually anyone can be helped.

What Does IV Sedation Involve?

This technique involves the use of a small cannula (needle) placed in the back of the hand or the arm through which a sedative is administered prior to treatment. Drug of choice is Midazolam, so it is extremely safe (although other drugs may be used if under the care of an anaesthetist).

As a patient, you are conscious the entire procedure, but don't let this put you off. You will experience an extremely relaxed state, to the point of drowsiness. Many patients are more than happy to take a nap during treatment. I should point out that IV sedation is not intended to put you to sleep or make you unconscious like a general anaesthetic. You just feel so relaxed and oblivious to your surroundings that you are happy to doze off. Because of this, time passes in what appears to be minutes, even when undertaking many hours of treatment.

IV sedation offers a significant number of benefits over that of oral sedation. First, it enables the dentist or anaesthetist to inject the sedative directly into the blood stream, which means a virtually instantaneous effect—you will start to feel the effects of the drug in less than thirty seconds. Second, a higher dose of drug can be safely used, enabling even the most anxious patient to be treated. Third, the drug can be topped up easily and frequently to maintain the level of sedation you need to stay comfortable.

Other benefits include a reduction in the gag reflex. Of greater significance is another side effect that may help you to manage your anxiety or phobia much better following treatment. Midazolam induces amnesia; it makes the majority of patients forget the entire experience. This benefit is appreciated by many patients, as generally the very anxious or phobic and do not want to remember.

There are some limitations to IV sedation. Those on medication and/or in poor health may not be suitable or find that treatment is not so effective. However, the main limitation is availability of the service. A significant number of dentists offer sedation dentistry throughout the UK, but many still do not. As a result, you may find you need to undertake treatment with a different dentist to gain the benefit of IV sedation.

General Anesthetic (GA)

General anaesthetic (GA) is very different than conscious sedation, IV sedation, and inhalation sedation. Under GA, you are completely unconscious, to the point that you feel no pain (even without local anaesthetic).

Virtually any dental treatment can be completed under GA, but there is a significantly higher risk of complications arising, in the worst-case even death. Because of this, GA is banned from general dental practice and can only be used in hospital under certain conditions.

Why Is GA Considered to Be a Risky Procedure?

GA induces complete unconsciousness, resulting in your inability to feel pain (great), but it also results in your inability to breathe for yourself (not so great). The assistance of an anaesthetist and a breathing tube are required to breathe for you, thus keeping you alive. Because of this, GA tends to place a strain on the heart and lungs, increasing post-treatment complications.

GA was withdrawn from general dental practice in 2000/2001. It was considered to be too dangerous following the tragic deaths of a number of patients, many of whom were children. Since then, all treatments requiring GA must be undertaken in hospital where superior resuscitation facilities are available.

Although GA may sound appealing to the very anxious or phobic, it is truly not the best way to undertake treatment. Why risk your life when you can undertake IV sedation, a treatment offering most of the benefits of GA but without the risks.

Additional Information

Due to the widespread nature of this problem (dental fear and anxiety), a significant amount of additional information is available online. Two such sites offering comprehensive information and a database of dentists offering treatment for anxious/fearful patients can be found at *www.dentalphobia.co.uk* and *www.dentalfearcentral.org*.

PART FIVE

ROLE OF THE SPECIALIST AND DENTAL TEAM

20

WHY YOU MAY CONSIDER THE HELP OF A SPECIALIST TO TRANSFORM YOUR SMILE OR DENTAL HEALTH

When choosing a particular dentist or considering a particular kind of treatment, you may find your treatment of choice falls within the sphere of care and services offered by a registered dental specialist, not just a general dental practitioner (GDP) with a special interest. It is important to note that there is a difference between the two.

A general dental practitioner can dedicate his or her career to a particular field of dentistry, undertaking post-graduate education to develop his or her knowledge and skills to the highest standards of care and best practice (e.g., implant dentistry). However, no matter how skilled the dentist is, he or she is not permitted to be called a specialist. He or she may only state that he or she holds a special interest in a particular field of dentistry.

To be recognised as a registered specialist in a particular field by the profession and GDC, a dentist must undertake an extensive training programme. This type of training programme meets criteria and learning objectives (both practical and academic) set by the GDC. This process takes years to complete under the supervision of specialist consultants within a teaching hospital environment.

The aim of this process is to help both the public and dental profession distinguish between those dentists proven to possess advanced skills and knowledge within a specific field of dentistry from those with a general knowledge-based background.

The General Dental Council classifies thirteen dental specialist areas. Of the thirteen specialties, only the first seven are of likely relevance, accessible by you the reader through self-referral in locations outside of a hospital environment. The remaining six specialties are beyond the scope of this book, where treatment would be received within a hospital environment or the community following referral from your general dentist. See *www.gdc-uk.org* for more information.

Prosthodontics

Endodontics

Periodontics

Restorative Dentistry

Oral Surgery

Orthodontics

Paediatric Dentistry

Special Care Dentistry *

Oral Medicine *

Dental Public Health *

Oral and Maxillofacial Pathology *

Dental and Maxillofacial Radiology *

Oral Microbiology *

* Indicates treatments normally offered within a hospital environment or the community, following referral to a specialist registered dentist or consultant.

Choosing Your Perfect Prosthodontist

Prosthodontist is the professional term used to describe a dentist specialising in the restoration of teeth, creating and placing natural-looking substitute or prosthetic teeth to restore an individual's mouth and smile back to health.

All dentists and registered dental specialists must possess a general knowledge of a wide range of dental procedures. Treatments considered to be a prosthodontist's area of expertise include:

- Aesthetic/Cosmetic dentistry
- Porcelain veneers
- Crowns and bridges
- Implant dentistry
- Complete and partial dentures
- Re-treatment of failing dentistry
- Tooth wear

The majority, if not all, of these treatments are often provided by GDPs (General Dental Practitioners) who have undertaken extensive postgraduate training to obtain the appropriate skills. The difference between a GDP and prosthodontist is that a prosthodontist has completed a rigorous formal training pathway recognised by the General Dental Council to meet set standards of care.

How Do You Know If You Need Treatment from a Prosthodontist?

Most of the time, you would probably visit a general dentist if you thought you had broken a tooth or filling or were in need of treatment for toothache.

You would consider seeking treatment from a prosthodontist when more extensive treatments are required, such as the treatment of extreme tooth wear, or replacement and aesthetic improvement of multiple teeth with crowns, bridges, and dental implants.

How Do You Find Your Perfect Prosthodontist?

There are two ways of seeking treatment with a prosthodontist. The first is via a referral from your existing dentist for treatment he or she has no experience in offering. Your existing dentist may recommend treatment with a prosthodontist for just one part of or all treatments you may require. For example, your dentist may ask a prosthodontist to complete surgery for a dental implant. Your existing dentist would then restore the implant with a new crown, thus providing you with a replacement tooth. Both the prosthodontist and your regular dentist would complete different parts of the treatment. Alternatively, your regular dentist may ask the prosthodontist to complete the entire procedure.

The second way to seek treatment is through a self-referral. You have the choice to go directly to a prosthodontist in the same manner you would choose to visit a general dentist, seeking recommendations from friends and family, or seeking advice and information from Internet sites like *www.MyPerfectDentist.com* or *www.CosmeticDentistryGuide. com*. The British Society for the Study of Prosthodontics at *www.bsspd. org* offers some additional information.

Choosing Your Perfect Endodontist

Endodontist is the professional term used to describe a dentist who specialises in providing root fillings. An endodontist deals specifically with the cause, diagnosis, prevention, and treatment of diseases and injuries of the tooth root, dental pulp (nerve), and surrounding tissue.

With information now readily available on the Web and in the media, most people have heard of the phrases "root filling," "root treatment," or "root canal." In its simplest form, root canal treatment involves the removal of the nerve from a tooth following irreversible damage from bacterial infection or trauma (injury). The resulting empty space within the tooth is then disinfected and filled with an internal rubber or plastic sealant known as a root filling.

Why Might You Need a Root Canal Filling?

Root canal treatment is an important tool employed by dentists for a number of reasons. The most important reason is to eliminate dental pain and infection without having to remove a tooth. Dental pain is a common problem, often caused by dental decay, fracture, or infection of a tooth due to injury to your teeth, whether accidental or deliberate. Root fillings may also be used electively (out of choice when no pain exists) to help repair an extensively damaged pain-free tooth or improve the appearance of a tooth with cosmetic dentistry.

If you experienced toothache before the introduction of root treatment procedures in the 1960s, the only way to solve the problem was to remove it. Nowadays dentistry offers treatments that can save the tooth.

How Do You Know If You Need a Root Filling?

In extreme cases, it is obvious if you need a root filling, as you will likely be experiencing severe toothache unable to be controlled with painkillers. You may find that your face becomes swollen and red, while the area will be painful to touch, signifying the formation of an abscess. You may also find that you feel unwell, often a result of running a temperature due to the infection.

However, the first indication of trouble may just be a noticeable increase in the sensitivity of a tooth to cold and hot drinks or foods, or breathing in cold air. This is often a sign that the nerve in a tooth is being irritated, probably by dental decay or a broken, worn out filling. If you notice this type of change within a single tooth, do not ignore it, as in most cases it will often lead to toothache. (Note: generalised tooth sensitivity to cold is often the result of excessive grinding of the teeth or gum recession.)

You may also find a root filling is recommended when undertaking routine dental treatment even when you have experienced no dental pain or sensitivity. It is not unusual for a dentist to find that when attempting to remove dental decay or repair a broken tooth or filling the nerve in the tooth will be damaged to the extent it will cause significant toothache after treatment. In this situation, the dentist will recommend a root filling as a preventive treatment.

Re-treatment of Old Root Fillings

If treated to the highest standards of care, a root filling will often last decades. However, sometimes root fillings do not work or break down prematurely, resulting in pain, swelling, and infection. Root fillings can never be guaranteed 100 percent successful, so failures do occur. In most cases, this can be rectified with re-treatment of the tooth by removing and replacing the old root filling.

I would always advise seeking the very best care possible if you require a root filling, especially if a root filling needs replacement. Root treatment is the foundation of your tooth, acting in a similar fashion to the foundation of a house. Just like a house, it does not matter what the house looks like; it will eventually collapse if the foundation is poor. Seeking treatment for a root filling with a specialised registered endodontist will offer you the best care and the best chance of long-term success. I routinely work with an endodontist providing a treatment success rate as high as 98 percent.

How Do You Find Your Perfect Endodontist?

There are two ways of seeking treatment from an endodontist. The first is via a referral from your existing dentist.

If you are in need of root treatment or re-treatment, your existing dentist may recommend treatment with an endodontist, or you may request a referral. Your dentist will normally know of an endodontist who can resolve the problems you are experiencing.

Again, you have the choice to self refer. Sources available to you when making this decision include asking friends and family and searching the Internet using *www.MyPerfectDentist.com* for a specialised registered endodontist. Another alternative is to visit the British Endodontic Society's Web site at *www.BritishEndodonticSociety.org.uk*. This society represents specialist registered endodontists in the UK and offers contact details for anyone seeking a self-referral.

My thanks to my colleague Dr. Alan Holland (GDC registered endodontic specialist at *www.RootFillings.com*) for his support and advice with this subject.

Choosing Your Perfect Periodontist

Periodontist is the professional term used to describe a dentist who specialises in the diagnosis, prevention, and treatment of gum disease and gum infection. Their expertise also includes gum surgery to aid dental health, cosmetic gum treatments associated with cosmetic dental procedures, and the replacement of missing teeth.

Why Might You Need Periodontal Treatment (Gum Therapy)?

Research indicates that around four out of every five people (80 percent of the population) will suffer from some level of gum disease at one point in their lifetime, and nearly one out of every ten people will suffer from advanced irreversible gum disease known as periodontitis. In its most severe form, periodontitis can result in the premature loss of some or all teeth.

Your gums are the foundation to your teeth and smile. Healthy gums are not only important for maintaining a healthy smile and keeping your teeth for life, but long-term research now indicates a strong link between gum disease and other general systemic illness of the body, including increased risk of fatal heart attack, stroke, diabetes, premature birth, rheumatoid arthritis, and more.

Why Do Some People Suffer from This Problem and Not Others?

Our knowledge is improving all the time of why this is. A number of major factors appear to be responsible. Family history, ethnicity, stress, and smoking are all important risk factors, while general diseases like diabetes increase an individual's susceptibility. Smoking is a significant risk factor in the development of gum disease. From just my own observations when treating patients, I can tell you that the vast majority of long-term smokers suffer from advanced irreversible gum disease resulting in the loss of most, if not all, of their teeth.

How Do You Know If You Need Periodontal Treatment (Gum Therapy)?

Gum disease rarely causes any pain until it has reached an advanced stage. This means most people infected with it do not know they have it until it is too late to treat or they start to lose teeth.

The signs and symptoms of gum disease vary from person to person. The main signs to look for are gums that bleed when brushing or spontaneous bleeding from the mouth, teeth that start to loosen or become wobbly, teeth that start to move (for example, you find that visible gaps start appearing between your teeth), and the development of bad breath (halitosis). The predominant cause of bad breath is the bacteria present in all of our mouths. It is those same bacteria that are also associated with the development of gum disease.

It is possible to be unaware of all these signs. It is therefore essential to attend a general dental practitioner regularly so that special assessment techniques, sometimes including X-rays, can be carried out as part of your routine dental health examinations. Early detection and treatment of this disease will not only prevent tooth loss, but it will also help reduce your risks of fatal heart attack, stroke, and many other systemic diseases now linked with gum infection.

How Do You Find Your Perfect Periodontist?

To become a recognised periodontist, a dentist must complete years of specialist training. In this case, choosing a periodontist will probably be quite different from choosing another specialist.

When choosing a cosmetic dentist or an orthodontist, you are aware of a condition or concern you have. For example, you are aware that you are unhappy with the appearance of your smile and you have made the decision to change it. Because gum disease causes no pain, it is often the case that you are completely unaware you even have a problem. It is therefore probable that you only become aware of this following a complete dental health check with a general dentist, or when visiting a specialist dentist for other types of treatment.

As with other dental specialties you may self refer using recommendations from friends and family, or using online listings found at *www.MyPerfectDentist.com.* You may also find the right periodontist for you through the British Society of Periodontology at *www.bsperio.org.uk.*

However, it is more likely that any referral will be through a general dentist following a diagnosis of gum disease. In many cases, a general dentist will be able to deal with early to intermediate gum disease, so a referral will probably not be necessary. Only when diagnosis of intermediate to advanced disease is confirmed are you likely to receive a referral to a periodontist.

If you find yourself in this unfortunate position, there is no reason that you cannot use the recommendations in this book to confirm that the periodontist your dentist recommends is perfect for you.

Choosing Your Perfect Restorative Dentist

Restorative dentist is the professional term used to describe a dentist specialising in the restoration of diseased, injured, or abnormal teeth back to normal function.

Unlike other dental specialties, specialist restorative dentists' expertise is multidisciplinary. They are recognised as offering specialist expert care in endodontics, periodontics, and prosthodontics.

You would choose to seek treatment, or be referred to a restorative dentist, if you possess multiple dental problems requiring many types of treatment to restore your dental health.

You will find your perfect restorative dentist in the same way as all other dental specialists discussed in this book, via a referral from your current dentist or by self-referral after researching the Internet and receiving recommendations from friends and family.

Choosing Your Perfect Surgical Dentist/Oral Surgeon

There is no official title describing a dentist who specialises in oral surgery. Two titles used within the profession are surgical dentist and oral surgeon. (Oral surgeon is sometimes used to describe a dentist holding a second qualification as a medic, practicing maxillofacial surgery within a hospital environment or surgical dentistry within private practice. Maxillofacial surgeons are governed by the General Medical Council.)

The General Dental Council's definition of a specialist dentist practicing oral surgery is "a dentist who deals with the treatment and ongoing management of irregularities and pathology of the jaw and mouth that require surgical intervention." This includes the specialty previously called surgical dentistry.

Basically, these are dentists recognised to have undertaken specialist training in dental treatments requiring surgical procedures, whether for disease, infection, or the replacement of missing teeth. They are not only experienced at working within the mouth but also outside the mouth and around the lips.

How Do You Know If You Need a Surgical Dentist/Oral Surgeon?

It is most likely that you would not know if you were in need of treatment from a surgical dentist/oral surgeon. If you found something abnormal like a lump in or around your mouth, or you experienced pain from wisdom teeth, you would most likely visit a general dentist or maybe even your local doctor. If in need of treatment, only then would you receive a referral to an oral surgeon.

Only when considering the replacement of missing teeth with dental implants or removing a problem tooth are you likely to consider the services of a general dentist or oral surgeon with surgical expertise.

How Do You Find Your Perfect Surgical Dentist/Oral Surgeon?

As previously mentioned, you are most likely to receive a referral to a registered specialist from your own general dentist, but you may also self refer for elective treatments considered to be more general, like the placement of dental implants or the removal of problematic wisdom teeth.

When self-referring, use recommendations from friends and family, or research the perfect dentist for you on a hosting site like *www. MyPerfectDentist.com*. A good resource if considering dental implant treatment is the Association of Dental Implantology (ADI) at *www.adi.*

org.uk. The British Association of Oral Surgeons may be searched online at www.baos.org.uk, but it provides little information to the public.

Choosing Your Perfect Orthodontist

Orthodontist is the professional term used to describe a dentist who specialises in providing orthodontic treatment, also known as braces. An orthodontist deals specifically with the development, prevention, and correction of irregularities of the teeth, bite, and jaw.

Why Might You Need Orthodontic Treatment (Braces)?

There are a number of reasons for using braces to correct the position of crooked teeth in both adults and children. The most obvious reason is to improve the appearance of a smile by straightening crooked, misaligned teeth into their correct position.

However, there are also a number of other reasons for undertaking treatment with an orthodontist for long-term dental health and well-being. Such reasons include: correction of a misaligned bite, correction of jaw growth in growing children, prevention of excessive tooth wear and irreversible damage to gums, reducing jaw joint problems and headaches, and helping in the replacement of missing teeth in combination with other dental treatments.

How Do You Know If You Need Orthodontic Treatment?

Orthodontic treatment is an obvious option and alternative to cosmetic dentistry (porcelain veneers and crowns) when considering the improvement of a crooked smile.

As an adult patient in particular, you may experience dental health issues that you never realised were attributed to crooked teeth and which could be fixed with the help of orthodontic treatment. Tooth clenching and grinding is a common problem experienced at night while sleeping by a majority of the population. For most people, they are unaware that they do it, and for many it is of little consequence.

Chronic clenching and grinding can often be attributed to an uneven bite. For a number of people, long-term clenching and grinding can result in jaw joint pain or clicking, teeth may become sensitive as a result of receding gums due to nighttime grinding, and clenching is a significant factor in the cause of tooth wear and even recurrent headaches. Depending how severe your uneven bite is, it is possible to reduce or eliminate the associated symptoms by realigning the way your teeth bite together using orthodontic treatment.

Movement and crowding of front teeth that were once straight can also be attributed to persistent clenching and grinding and an uneven bite. Long-term clenching and grinding causes tooth wear. Your body will adapt to this by allowing your teeth to move over time and compensate for this wear. In most cases, this process occurs over many years with teeth drifting toward the front of the mouth. The net result: crooked front teeth that were once perfectly straight.

How Do You Find Your Perfect Orthodontist?

To become a recognised orthodontist, a dentist must complete years of specialist training. As with other dental specialties, you may request a referral from your regular dentist, or your dentist may recommend orthodontic treatment if he feels it will be of benefit to you.

Alternatively, you may self refer, choosing the right orthodontist for you via recommendations from friends and family. Again, an excellent source of information is available online, where you can find a specialist registered orthodontist at *www.MyPerfectDentist.com*, as well as through the orthodontist professional association, the British Orthodontic Society *www.bos.org.uk*.

Choosing Your Children's Perfect Dentist (General or Paediatric Dentist)

Children's dentistry is most often provided by general dentists, but specialist children's dentists exist. Paediatric dentist is the professional term used to describe a dentist who specialises in the treatment of children. Paediatric dentists provide both general and specialist dental care for children and adolescence. They are based within hospitals or the community, working as part of a comprehensive team including orthodontists and oral surgeons to help children with a range of dental problems. This includes caring for those who demonstrate intellectual, psychological, and/or emotional problems, as well as medical and physical ones.

Why Is It Important for Your Child to See a Dentist?

There are two primary reasons for having your children's teeth examined by a dentist. The first is to check their general dental health and well-being so that their teeth grow correctly; the second is to deal with the all-too-common problem of dental trauma.

The needs of a growing child will always differ from that of an adult patient. When treating children, a dentist is not only looking to check for correct growth and development, but he or she also manages current problems as well as anticipates any future problems that may arise in a child's development. It is often a surprise to parents to find out that their child's dentition will not completely mature until their late teens or early twenties, with wisdom teeth erupting and growth still occurring on average until twenty-one years of age.

As a concerned parent, it is important that your child's teeth are examined at least once a year from about two-and-a-half years of age until adulthood. More often than not, your dentist would expect to see very little out of the ordinary, but it is important to detect any signs of dental decay or abnormally growing or missing teeth early.

As a dentist with a special interest in cosmetic and implant dentistry, I see very few children, but at a time when I did, I encountered a common misconception from parents. Many parents assume incorrectly that it does not matter if their child's milk teeth (baby teeth) are a cause for concern, as these will be replaced in time by adult teeth. Unfortunately, this misunderstanding results in many children experiencing dental treatment at a young age that could have been prevented if dealt with earlier on. This not only exposes children to treatment at a young age that can leave them traumatised for life, but dental negligence can have long-lasting effects on the developing adult dentition. For example, early loss of a milk tooth due to dental decay can result in the space for the adult tooth being lost. The result of this will be the need for braces as a teenager to recreate the previously lost space or accept crooked teeth.

Dental Trauma (Accidental Injury)

Dental decay is still the number one cause of childhood dental problems. Secondary to this is dental trauma. Research indicates that it is not uncommon for children to damage their baby or adult teeth through accidental injury.

What do you do if your child accidentally damages his or her new front adult teeth? The first thing is not to panic; things often look worse than they are. The next step is to take your child to see a dentist as soon as possible. If you see that a tooth has been chipped or knocked out entirely, try to find it and place it in a container of milk. If treated within one hour, it may be possible to put the tooth back.

If a dentist is not available—for example, it is late at night or you are miles from home—then find the nearest hospital accident and emergency department. They will normally have a dentist available on call to deal with emergencies involving dental trauma. Please note, this service is not designed to deal with general dental problems like toothache; it is for traumatic emergencies only!

How Do You Find Your Children's Perfect Dentist?

More often than not you will take your child to see a general dentist. Most general dentists will offer dentistry for children, but some do not, not because they are not qualified to do so, but because their interests are in other areas.

As most general dentists offer children's dentistry, the best way to assess the most appropriate dentist for your child is to research them in the same way you would for yourself. Again, you may ask friends and family, or you may find Web sites like *www.MyPerfectDentist.com* most useful.

Self-referral to a paediatric dentist is possible, but more often than not your child will only receive care from a paediatric dentist via a referral from a general dentist, as they are normally based in hospitals. A Web site for the British Society of Paediatric dentistry does exist at *www. bspd.co.uk;* however, this is intended for professional use only and does not list specialist paediatric dentists.

The Role of the General Dental Practitioner (a General Dentist or GDP)

The vast majority of registered dentists in the UK, including myself, are considered to be General Dental Practitioners (GDPs) holding the qualification of BDS (Bachelor of Dental Science) or the equivalent. This qualification entitles a dentist to register with the GDC (General Dental Council) and perform all those treatments considered to be part of general dental practice, like the filling and removal of teeth. This qualification also entitles general dentists to offer treatments a registered dental specialist can offer so long as they are competent to do so.

In practice, this means a general dentist can offer treatments normally thought exclusive to a dental specialist. Therefore, as a general dentist I can remove teeth and offer my patients fillings, but I can also offer orthodontic treatment (braces) or complete complex oral surgery, as long as I have completed the appropriate training.

As a perspective patient searching for your perfect dentist, you may find that a general dentist possesses the appropriate experience necessary to complete the treatment you require. Good examples of this are with cosmetic and implant dentistry. There are no recognised specialist qualifications for either of these fields of dentistry, so you will find that many general dentists offer these treatments as well as registered specialist dentists like prosthodontists, periodontists, and restorative dentists.

You may find that a general dentist who has dedicated his or her entire career to a particular field of dentistry may actually possess a greater level of experience than a registered specialist dentist.

It is of no surprise then that making a decision can become very confusing. So, how do you decide between a general dentist and registered specialist dentist?

You should use this book, the many recommendations I have mentioned, as well as the fifteen questions you must ask before choosing your perfect dentist to help with your decision.

21

DENTAL CARE PROFESSIONALS (DCPS)— WHO ARE THEY AND WHAT DO THEY DO?

Dental Care professionals, or DCPs, as they are commonly known, are the highly skilled individuals who collectively form the "dental team," supporting dentists in the delivery of care to patients on a daily basis.

All DCPs are legally required to be registered with the General Dental Council in the same manner as a dentist and are classified as:

- Dental Nurses
- Dental Hygienists
- Dental Therapists
- Orthodontic Therapists
- Dental Technicians
- Clinical Dental Technicians

Dental Nurses

Dental nurses, also known as dental assistants, are one of the most important but commonly undervalued members of the dental team, and without which a dentist and dental practice cannot function. They work with and under the direction of a dentist to perform a number of important duties, which include:

- Working with the dentist to provide active dental care to patients

- Understanding all dental procedures along with all instruments and materials involved, whether this be extensive surgery to place dental implants or a standard filling

- A comprehensive knowledge and maintenance of cross infection control and sterilisation of instruments for patient safety

- A knowledge of first aid in case of medical emergencies

- Setting up and cleaning down of surgeries so treatments can actually take place

In addition to these critical roles, many nurses are also qualified to take X-rays and offer oral health education directly to patients. They may also be trained to perform basic dental laboratory techniques like that of a dental technician.

Dental Hygienists

Dental hygienists work under the direction of a dentist to provide clinical and educational care to help patients achieve and maintain good oral health. Dental hygienists focus on the treatment and prevention of gum disease, and cleaning and removing the hard deposits on teeth known as tartar (or calculus). Tartar is the hard calcium deposits that develop above and below the gum line, promoting gum disease that cannot be removed with a toothbrush. This is a much more complex and skilled procedure than people realise and takes years of training to perform correctly.

Dental hygienists are also trained in the prevention of dental decay and non-invasive cosmetic treatments. Under direction of a dentist, they may perform additional treatments, including tooth whitening, taking of X-rays, placement of temporary fillings, and preventive care (treatments designed to reduce the chance of dental disease developing).

Preventive care includes the placement of fissure sealants (a protective plastic coating painted on to the tooth surface) and topical fluoride (a fluoride varnish painted onto teeth that possess a higher susceptibility to tooth decay).

Hygienists are an invaluable part of a modern dental practice, enabling dentists to offer the best dental care available.

Dental Therapists

Dental therapists are a relatively new addition to the dental team. Their role is similar to that of a dental hygienist, working under direction of a dentist to provide clinical and educational care to help patients achieve and maintain good oral health.

Importantly, they have undertaken additional training and are qualified to complete more complex treatments, such as fillings, for both adults and children. They are also qualified to perform a range of other treatments on children's teeth (known as deciduous or "milk teeth"). These treatments include the placement of pre-formed crowns, pulp/nerve treatments, and the removal of deciduous teeth under local anaesthetic.

Importantly, both hygienists and dental therapists are trained to recognise a range of dental diseases, including oral cancer and tooth decay, so that they may inform and refer patients back to their dentist for the appropriate care and treatment.

Orthodontic Therapists

Like dental therapists, orthodontic therapists are a new addition to the dental team. In a similar fashion to dental therapists, orthodontic therapists are qualified to support orthodontists in the provision of orthodontic treatments (braces). Orthodontic therapists are trained to fit and maintain orthodontic appliances under the direction of a dentist.

Dental Technicians

Dental technicians are the highly skilled and creative individuals responsible for crafting the very best custom-made porcelain veneers, crowns, and dentures used by cosmetic dentists, implant dentists, and general dentists to enhance a patient's smile and replace missing teeth.

Many people think that their dentist is responsible for creating their crowns or porcelain veneers when undertaking treatment. More often than not this is not the case, but in some cases this is true.

I am a cosmetic dentist, but I am also dual qualified as a dental technician. I trained as a dental technician for seven years, specialising in cosmetic dentistry and dental implants before returning to university for an additional five years.

What advantages does this experience offer me? This enables me to complete the entire treatment process from start to finish. It provides me with complete control over the quality and care I offer my patients. I possess a unique perspective when working with other technicians to complete my patients' treatments to the highest standards. I am just one of a small percentage of dentists to have trained in this way in the UK.

With advancement in technology, such as computer-aided design systems (CADCAM), dentists can now create restorations like veneers and crowns without having to undertake many years of additional training as a dental technician. However, the final results are still dependent on the dentist's artistic ability and technical skill to create the most natural-looking porcelain veneers and crowns. Again, the number of dentists able to provide the highest standards of treatment and care in this fashion without the creative and artistic ability of a dental technician is limited.

It takes many years and dedication to train as a dental technician. Just like dentists, there are those technicians who specialise in offering the highest quality cosmetic and restorative treatments, and there are those who do not. For the very best treatment results, your dentist needs to work with a dental technician of the highest calibre.

When your dentist mentions that he will be sending your crowns and veneers to the laboratory, he means your tooth or teeth will be created by a dental technician. If you are lucky, you may choose a dentist with a dental laboratory in the same building as the practice. Advantages of an on-site laboratory are that the dental technician can assess your teeth at the same time as the dentist. The technician can examine your smile in person, while you describe exactly what you are looking for. This will help the technician make your crowns and veneers look the very best possible and ultimately make your smile look exactly how you want it.

When choosing a dentist and undertaking any type of treatment requiring laboratory-made porcelain veneers, crowns, bridges and dentures, you are perfectly in your rights to ask the dentist which technician or laboratory he intends to use. You can then research the technician to determine if he or she meets your requirements.

Clinical Dental Technicians

Clinical dental technicians are also able to create custom-made porcelain veneers, crowns, and dentures used by cosmetic, implant, and general dentists to treat their patients.

However, they have also undertaken additional training (in a similar fashion to a dental therapist) to provide treatment directly to a patient as part of the dental team. In particular, clinical dental technicians are qualified to create and provide removable dentures directly to patients.

As the majority of clinical dental technicians work within their own practices, they are also qualified to recognise a range of dental diseases, including oral cancer and tooth decay, so that they may inform and refer patients to a dentist for the appropriate care and treatment.

22

WHAT DO THE
LETTERS STAND FOR?

By Dr. Neil Gerrard and Dr. Bertrand Napier

In the UK, dentists will generally have the letters BDS (Bachelor of Dental Surgery) or BChD or LDS (Licentiate in Dental Surgery) after their name. Universities award degrees, whereas the royal colleges award licences and diplomas. Thus, the basic qualification awarded on graduation is either the BDS or BChD degree, or the LDS licence from one of the colleges.

Many dental practitioners will have both qualifications, since both examinations may have been taken as undergraduates, but note that these qualifications are of equal standing and thus provide no indication of a higher degree of training or expertise than in the case of those individuals who hold only one.

Some foreign graduates may have other letters after their name (e.g., DDS for North America). These are different letters that generally mean the same thing: a qualified dentist.

Higher Qualifications

The dentist may also have other letters after his or her name, which indicates a postgraduate qualification.

Universities award higher degrees to dentists who have undergone recognised (and usually rigorous) postgraduate courses of study or research, followed by examination or the submission of a thesis. These will be master's degrees (MSc, MDS, or MPhil) or doctorates (PhD or very rarely, DSc). While these are positive indicators of an individual's intellect, they do not always indicate *clinical* expertise. For example, the MPhil or PhD (Master or Doctor of Philosophy) degrees will in all probability be awarded on the strength of a *research project* and are an unreliable indication of the standard of *practical expertise* of the holder.

Mastership in Clinical Dentistry (MClinDent) is a postgraduate degree offered by universities consisting of both academic and clinical assessment. Although MCinDent does not qualify a dentist to be placed on the specialist register, it does indicate a high level of practical and theoretical training in a specific field of dentistry.

Royal colleges award diplomas to dentists who have undertaken recognised and approved postgraduate courses of study, followed by formal examinations that usually have both written and practical elements. These awards will be diplomas, such as the DDPH (Diploma in Dental Public Health), memberships, such as the MFGDP (UK) and the MGDS, or fellowships, such as the FDS (Fellowship in Dental Surgery).

The MFGDP (UK) and the MGDS give an indication that they have studied general dental practice beyond the basic qualification level, the MGDS being the senior qualifications. However, be advised that initially some of these were awarded without examination, on a "grandfathering" basis, so possession of this diploma does not necessarily mean that the holder has been tested by his or her peers in open examination.

The MJDF RCSEng is a new qualification developed by the Faculty of Dental Surgery of the Royal College of Surgeons of England and the Faculty of General Dental Practice (UK). This qualification intends to progressively replace the existing MFDS and MFGDP.

FFGDP indicates fellowship of the Faculty of General Dental Practice (UK). This qualification represents the culmination of many years of study in general dental practice and follows MFGDP and the newer MJDF, thus marking the end of a career pathway.

In all cases, neither the MFGDP (UK), the MGDS, the newer MJDF, or the higher qualification of FFDGP indicate specialist knowledge or training.

Practitioners will also be encountered who have undergone postgraduate education in the United States, usually leading to the award of master's degrees, MSc (Master of Science) or MS (Master of Surgery). These qualifications invariably indicate a high standard of postgraduate training.

Accreditation or Fellowship Status

There are various associations nationally and internationally offering educational pathways for their member dentists. These educational pathways normally involve a rigorous examination process leading to a recognisable achievement within the association (e.g., Accreditation or Fellowship status).

It should be noted that these achievements are only recognised by the association in question and are not an academic qualification. Although not formally recognised as a specialist qualification by the GDC (General Dental Council), these examinations are designed to test both the theoretical and practical knowledge of the participating dentist to the highest clinical standards. Any dentist achieving this recognition may be considered to possess expert knowledge in the area of practice the association represents.

Other *"Qualifications"*

A number of independent "educational institutes" have developed postgraduate courses for dentists, both within the UK and abroad (particularly North America). Many of these centers offer modular courses, which often bestow a title or a level of achievement upon the participating dentist when completed. Examples of these are dentists stating they have "graduated" or have achieved a "master's level" from a particular institute's programme. These titles are not recognised academic qualifications and should not be confused with master's degrees offered by universities. They also offer no indication of specialist training, neither are they recognised by the General Dental Council

(GDC). However, they can infer a commitment by the dentist to quality continuing education in an area of special interest.

Some dentists also have commitments with the administrative and political bodies of the profession. Valuable as these are to the dental community, it should be recognised that membership, for example, of an LDC (Local Dental Committee), says nothing about that individual's clinical expertise and/or training.[7]

---

7 This information has been reprinted with the kind permission of the British Academy of Cosmetic Dentistry (BACD) www.bacd.com.

PART SIX

RESOLVING PROBLEMS

23

WHAT IF THINGS GO WRONG?

The primary aim of this book is to provide you with the knowledge you need to make the right choice when choosing a new dentist. If you have taken the time and effort to follow my advice and research the perfect dentist for you, you should not find yourself in the position of being dissatisfied with the treatment and service you have received, or find any subsequent need to make a complaint.

Unfortunately, life is never that simple, and things can and do go wrong. Whether a particular type of treatment has failed prematurely or resulted in additional problems, or the service received has fallen short of your expectations, you may feel a complaint is justified.

Some of the Most Common Complaints Relate To:

- Complications following treatment
- Communication
- Treatment charges
- Handling of complaints

24

COMPLICATIONS
FOLLOWING TREATMENT

Complications following dental treatment do arise and cannot always be predicted. In both dentistry and medicine, public expectations can be high. People have a tendency to expect modern dental treatments to be 100 percent successful 100 percent of the time, and patients are quick to apportion blame when failures occur.

Failures may indeed occur due to inappropriate of substandard care, but for the vast majority of cases failures occur unpredictably following treatments that have been successfully performed by a dentist hundreds, if not thousands, of times. Very often the reason a procedure may be successful 99 percent of the time, but fail for one in every hundred patients, is because we are all different.

Essentially we are all biologically the same, but small variations in our DNA result in an infinite number of subtle differences. For example, everyone's teeth are slightly different in size, shape, and colour, while some people chew harder on their teeth than others. A dentist will therefore use all of his experience to compensate for these variations, but still, some variations fall outside of "normal" and fail. It is also important to note that as with many areas of medicine, science still fails to offer us all the answers.

What Should You Do if Treatment Fails?

If you find yourself in the unfortunate position of failing treatments or complications, then the first thing you should do is contact your dentist. Any dentist with a good reputation will stand by his or her treatment and will often be more than willing to resolve any problem you are experiencing. The very best dentists will offer something akin to a warranty; for example, I offer a five-year promise on all cosmetic porcelain veneers or crowns and fillings, and I will replace them whatever the cause of failure within this time. All I ask is that you the patient undertake regular hygiene and dental health examinations. (It is important you understand that some treatments can never be guaranteed due to the nature of the treatment or the uniqueness of a patient's particular circumstance.)

If you have returned to your dentist but find that your experience is still less than satisfactory, then you need to consider what to do next—whether this entails additional treatment, if required, or filing a formal complaint if your experience really has been left wanting.

25

COMMUNICATION

Many complaints arise due to a lack of communication, either before, during, or after treatment, rather than a deliberate attempt to mislead or withhold information. In many situations where a complaint has arisen, the dentist has failed to understand a patient's requirements and expectations from the outset. However, a lack of communication is not just the sole preserve of the dentist. Patients possess little or no dental knowledge, so understandably many patients find it hard to communicate their exact requirements and expectations prior to treatment.

So How Do You Improve Communication with Your Chosen Dentist?

When considering a particular type of dental procedure, such as cosmetic dentistry or orthodontic braces, it is worth reflecting on what you are trying to achieve and what your ideal smile would look like at the end of treatment. An experienced dentist will be skilled at helping you decide what your ultimate goal is, but attending your first consultation prepared will enable you to communicate your thoughts and feelings much more effectively and thus reduce the chance of miscommunication. I often provide my patients with a questionnaire. This helps focus people's thoughts while providing me with useful information. If this type of questionnaire is not provided by your chosen dentist, then write a list of key notes and take it with you.

It is important that you are honest about your expectations during your consultation. For example, if you are fearful of treatment, it is important to discuss this, as your dentist is then more likely to offer you something you actually want, like sedation dentistry, rather than what he or she thinks you want. If considering cosmetic dentistry, are you looking for a completely new smile or the smile you used to have? It is also helpful to the dentist if you can describe what you currently like about your own smile and specifically what you don't like. You may find this uncomfortable and embarrassing, but I promise you the majority of dentists have heard the same concerns many times before and will not judge you in any way.

Ask the dentist to repeat back to you an explanation of your concerns and long-term goals. A simple question along the following lines is all that is needed: "Now that I have explained the way I feel about my dental health and smile, would you mind summarising this in your own words so I feel confident you understand me?" No ethical dentist would be offended by this question. In this way, you will be able to judge if he or she has listened and understood you correctly. If not, outline your concerns again until you are happy that the dentist understands exactly what you are looking for.

It is important that you choose a dentist with experience in the field of dental treatment you are looking to undertake. The dentist should not only possess the technical knowledge to provide the very best dental care, but he or she should also possess the skills and experience necessary to understand your requirements.

To Summarise:

- Try to have a clear idea of what you are looking for before attending a consultation (if you are not sure, write a list of concerns and take it with you).

- Answer all questions as honestly as possible, as the dentist needs to understand exactly what you want.

- Ask the dentist to explain your expectations in his or her own words.

- Choose a dentist with experience of the treatment you are interested in.

26

TREATMENT CHARGES

Misunderstandings relating to treatment costs are a surefire way to create distrust between a patient and dentist and will often result in a complaint. No one likes to be presented with a bill for a specific type of treatment only to be told that it is more than he or she was originally quoted.

I go to great lengths to outline all treatments and costs to my patients before I even start dental treatment. I will always try to cover all eventualities so that that there are no surprises, whether it is with treatment procedures or the costs involved.

An experienced dentist will possess an accurate idea of what to expect during treatment; however, due to anatomical variations, dentists will never truly know what they will encounter until they physically treat a tooth. Sometimes there is no option but to perform additional unexpected treatments leading to unexpected costs. In this situation, I would always cease treatment, explain my findings, and seek my patient's approval before continuing further.

What Should You Do to Prevent Unexpected Treatment Charges?

As a patient, you should expect and request a comprehensive treatment plan of any proposed treatments as well as the costs involved. It is important at this stage that you understand and are completely happy with proposed treatments and costs; if you are unsure in any way, inform the dentist of your concerns. As a dentist, I am happy to answer as many questions as my patients feel they need to ask.

Note: there is no such thing as a stupid or dumb question. If you do not understand something, keep asking questions until you are completely satisfied.

To Summarise:

- Always request a treatment plan outlining costs and treatment.

- Make sure you understand all costs and treatment procedures before undertaking treatment.

- Ask as many questions as you need to feel satisfied you are making the correct decision.

- If any of this information is not forthcoming, then reconsider treatment or find another dentist.

27

HANDLING OF COMPLAINTS

A significant number of official complaints by patients to the various complaint handling services derive from the frustration and inability of a disappointed patient to achieve recognition of his or her concerns. A secondary complaint arises that the original complaint was not dealt with satisfactorily.

The best advice I can offer is to avoid this situation in the first place by:

- Being realistic about your treatment goals (don't expect impossible miracles)

- Making sure your chosen dentist understands exactly what you are looking for through open communication

- Making sure you clearly understand the costs and treatments involved before proceeding with treatment

So What Should You Do and Expect if Service and Quality of Care Failed to Meet Your Expectations and a Complaint Is Justified?

Please note: The following information is intended for those with legitimate complaints who fail to resolve disagreements through local resolution. Unfortunately, a very small number of "rogue" dentists tarnish the hard work and genuine commitment of the entire dental profession (both NHS and private dentistry alike).

119

Without doubt, these individuals deserve to be prosecuted and lose their license to practice. However, the UK has now become the second most litigious country in the world for claims against dentists, surprisingly ranking even higher than the United States (the highest being Hong Kong).[8] This is a worrying trend that appears to be affecting society at large and more suggestive of the times we live in rather than the quality of UK dentistry.

Although the following information discusses the procedures you should follow when pursuing an unresolved complaint, I do not advocate the persistent appealing of decisions that have failed to fall in favour of the complainant. If you find yourself in a position where your complaint has been rejected, not just by the dentist, but one of the complaints services as well, then it may be time to reassess your position.

If service and quality of care has failed to meet your expectations and you feel you have a legitimate reason to complain, how should you proceed with your complaint to reach a quick and satisfactory resolution?

I recommend you follow the pathway depicted in the flow chart on the next page:

---

8 Data supplied by Dental Protection.

Step 1.
Local resolution
with your dentist

Step 2.
Dental Complaints
Service for private
dental care

Step 2.
NHS complaints
service for NHS
dental care

Step 3.
Referral to the General
Dental Council by
Complaints Services if a
conduct and behaviour issue

Step 4.
Take legal action
against dentist

28

LOCAL RESOLUTION

First of all, you should always bring your concerns to the attention of the dentist or staff members you received treatment or service from. In general, dentists and dental care professionals want their patients to be happy with their treatment and will do everything they can to resolve a problem or shortcoming that results in a complaint.

Whether your dentist offers private or NHS dental care, he or she will have a high-quality dental complaints procedure conforming to GDC (General Dental Council) guidelines. These procedures are designed to reassure and protect you the patient as a member of the general public.

You may wish to inform your dentist of your concerns verbally or through a letter. Most people feel uncomfortable making a verbal complaint, so writing your thoughts and concerns in the form of a letter is a good way of communicating your disappointments. A letter will enable you to list all of your concerns in a nonconfrontational manner, making it less likely for you to forget any points you wish to make. Another advantage of a letter is that the dentist in question has time to reflect on the points you are making objectively before replying to your concerns. You are much more likely to find the dentist sympathetic to your situation if he has time to imagine himself in your shoes, rather than reacting to a verbal confrontation. Remember, dentists are only human, and no one likes to be criticised. Verbal confrontation has a tendency to make everyone defensive; the result further strains the patient-dentist relationship, leading to an outcome that benefits no one.

It is also a good idea to let the dentist know the outcome you are looking for and what he or she can do to resolve your complaint. For example, are you looking for a simple apology and acknowledgment that your concerns were taken seriously, or are you looking for additional treatment to resolve a problem tooth, or do you feel you deserve your money back? Dentists are not mind readers, so telling them how they can resolve the problem can help them quickly meet your expectations.

As a patient, you should expect your complaint to be answered within a timely fashion. GDC guidelines indicate you should receive a reply within five working days, the NHS within three working days. However, offering the dentist a little more time—such as seven to ten working days—will allow the dentist time to consider your position, while expecting an immediate answer may result in a snap response.

If you receive a reply that meets your expectations, then great. If not, what do you do next? It really depends on the reply. You may receive a reply offering a compromise that, upon reflection, you find acceptable or offers room for negotiation. If so, keep communicating with your dentist until a satisfactory arrangement is achieved. If you receive a reply that you feel is completely unsatisfactory, or no reply at all, then you may wish to pursue your complaint further.

So What Do You Do Next to Take Your Complaint Higher?

You have a number of avenues available to pursue your complaint further if you are unable to resolve your differences in house (through local resolution/direct communication with the dentist and dental practice). These include the Dental Complaints Service for private dental care and the NHS complaints service (through your NHS dentist and local primary care trust) for NHS dental care. Finally, you may wish to take legal advice and pursue legal action through the courts.

The GDC (General Dental Council) also deals with complaints relating to the conduct and behaviour of all dental care professionals.

29

DENTAL COMPLAINTS SERVICE

For private dental care, the Dental Complaints Service should be your first point of call. They act to mediate between patient and dentist, offering a free impartial service to all patients receiving private dental care.

The Dental Complaints Service (DCS) will take your complaint seriously. They will listen to your point of view and all the circumstances leading up to your complaint. They will also look at the dentist's point of view as well as the outcome of any treatment you received. If you are unable to resolve your disagreement with the help of DCS, you and the dentist will be invited to attend a DCS panel meeting. Once the panel has examined all the particulars of your case, they will present a recommendation either supporting your complaint or not.

If they support your complaint, they will expect the dentist to accept their decision and comply with any recommendations they make, whether this be a simple apology, refund of fees, a contribution toward remedial work, or recommendations for future practice. Any recommendations the Dental Complaints Service make are not legally binding, and a dentist is under no legal obligation to follow them. However, it is unlikely any dentists will ignore their recommendations, because if they do, they are likely to be judged harshly if the complaint reaches the GDC (General Dental Council) and the complaint is found to be of merit.

If you find yourself in need of help with mediation relating to private dental treatment, you may contact the Dental Complaints Service online at *www.DentalComplaints.org.uk* or by telephone at: 08456 120 540.

I would like to acknowledge the assistance of Rachel Knight and the Dental Complaints Service with delivery of this information.

30

NHS COMPLAINTS SERVICE

Complaints procedures vary for NHS health and dental services throughout the UK. Outlined below are the different procedures operated by England, Scotland, Wales, and Northern Ireland. Please note: given the time lapse between writing and publishing, it is impossible for a book to be perfectly current; you may therefore encounter procedures that have been updated since first publication of this book.

NHS Complaints Services for England

For NHS dental care in England, the NHS complaints service will be your first point of call. All NHS dental services are commissioned locally through your PCT (Primary Care Trust). Any dentist working within the NHS will therefore be answerable to your local PCT, and any complaints relating to NHS dental care will be dealt with and through your PCT if you are unable to resolve your complaint directly with the dentist.

All NHS dentists should have a robust complaints procedure meeting standards set by your PCT and GDC. If you wish to pursue a complaint regarding NHS dentistry, you should follow the information your NHS dentist is obliged to provide you. This will outline your options and the step-by-step procedure your complaint will take. If for some reason you are unable to obtain this information, then you may make a complaint directly to your PCT via the NHS complaints service. This can be found online at *www.nhs.uk.*

A number of other avenues are also available to NHS patients, which include:

- The Patient Advice and Liaison Service (PALS) available in all hospitals

- The Independent Complaints Advocacy Service (ICAS), a national service that may be contacted through PALS

- The Parliamentary and Health Service Ombudsman (who are independent of the NHS and government); to contact call: 0345 015 4033

- NHS Direct (for England only) can also advise on NHS complaints; call 0845 4647

NHS Complaints Services for Scotland

For NHS dental care in Scotland, you should file your complaint with your local health board if you fail to resolve your dispute directly with your dentist.

In addition to this, you may file a complaint with the Scottish Public Services Ombudsman if resolution of your complaint through your local health board is unsatisfactory (although it should be noted that the ombudsman is not obliged to investigate every complaint).

Contact details for filing complaints in Scotland are listed at the end of the book

NHS Complaints Services for Wales

For NHS dental care in Wales, you should file your complaint with your local health board if you fail to resolve your dispute directly with your dentist.

In addition to this, you may file a complaint with the Health Service Ombudsman of Wales if resolution of your complaint through your local health board is unsatisfactory (although it should be noted that the ombudsman is not obliged to investigate every complaint).

Contact details for filing complaints in Wales are listed at the end of the book.

NHS Complaints Service for Northern Ireland

For NHS dental care in Northern Ireland, you should file your complaint with the Health and Social Care board for your local area if you fail to resolve your dispute directly with your dentist.

In addition to this, you may file a complaint with the Northern Ireland Ombudsman if resolution of your complaint through your local Health and Social Care Board is unsatisfactory (although it should be noted that the ombudsman is not obliged to investigate every complaint).

Contact details for filing complaints in Northern Ireland are listed at the end of the book.

31

THE GDC
(GENERAL DENTAL COUNCIL)

The GDC is charged with policing the entire dental profession (which includes all dental care professionals). Their primary objective is to deal with issues affecting a dentist's fitness to practice. This includes professional conduct and behaviour, health of the individual, as well as the individual's performance.

Everyone feels justified in his or her complaint; however, if your complaint is that you were overcharged for dental treatment by £50, then a complaint service equipped to deal with this type of issue in a prompt, efficient manner will serve you better—for example, the Dental Complaints Service for private dental care or the NHS complaints for all dental care provided under the NHS.

Mediation through these services should always be your first point of call failing local resolution of your complaint with your dentist. If they are unable to assist due to the nature of the complaint or feel your complaint is of a serious nature (conduct or behaviour issue), they may forward your complaint to the GDC for further investigation.

Further information about the GDC and its role in the regulation of the dental profession is available online at *www.gdc-uk.org*.

32

TAKE LEGAL ACTION—
A WORD OF WARNING!

Some patients feel it necessary to take direct legal action against a dentist, and in some cases this may be justified. As a patient, you may be left with no alternative but to take legal action if you have exhausted all other avenues of mediation. You have only to look online to find a number of solicitors specialising in dental malpractice offering help, claiming to recover your money and win you compensation for a no-win no-fee deal.

Beware, a word of warning! Use these services as the very last resort, not a first point of call. On more than one occasion, I have been in contact with patients seeking second opinions and treatment to correct failing dentistry. On all occasions, I have suggested that these patients seek a refund directly from the dentist for a quick resolution or use the available complaints services to mediate on their behalf. Unfortunately, these patients have found themselves in a state of uncertainty, unable to deal directly with their original dentist or resolve their concerns through the appropriate complaints services.

And the reason for this? These patients made the mistake of taking legal action before considering the alternatives. They did not seek impartial mediation through the Dental Complaints Service for private dental care or local NHS complaints service for NHS dental care. What they did do was contact those solicitors specialising in dental malpractice and as a consequence have found themselves tied into legal contracts committing them to the pursuit of a financial claim against their previous dentist.

If they decide at any point to drop the claim, then they find themselves liable for all legal costs they have incurred to date and so feel obligated to continue. Now, it is likely they will receive a refund and possibly some form of compensation (solicitors will only take cases they feel they have a good chance of winning), but more often than not it takes many months and in some cases years before a settlement is agreed.

If you wish to avoid the stresses associated with this situation, follow the advice I offer in this book. There is a good chance you will be able to settle your complaint in a relatively short span of time and to complete satisfaction without involving the services of a solicitor.

Citizens Advice Bureau

Finally, the Citizens Advice Bureau is always available to help with advice. For England, Wales, and Northern Ireland they can be contacted online at *www.CitizensAdvice.org.uk*. For Scotland, go to *www.cas.org.uk.*

Contact details for Northern Ireland Health and Social Care Board and Northern Ireland Ombudsman are:

Call your local care board at 0800 665544 or online at *www.n-i.nhs.uk.*

Alternatively, contact the central office at:
12-22 Linenhall Street
Belfast,
BT2 8BS
028 9043 4004

Northern Ireland Ombudsman
Northern Ireland Ombudsman
33 Wellington Place
Belfast
BT1 6HN
www.ni-ombudsman.org.uk

Contact details for Scottish local health boards and Scottish Public Services Ombudsman are:

To find contact details for your local NHS Board:
look in the phone book under "health services"
call the NHS Helpline at 0800 22 44 88
(textphone 18001 0800 22 44 88), or
look online at *www.hris.org.uk* or
www.show.scot.nhs.uk/organisations/orgindex.htm

Scottish Public Services Ombudsman
The Scottish Public Services Ombudsman
Freepost EH641
Edinburgh
EH3 0BR

Phone: 0800 377 7330
Fax: 0800 377 7331
Text message: 07900 494 372
E-mail: ask@spso.org.uk
www.spso.org.uk

Scotland—NHS 24
NHS 24 is a twenty-four-hour telephone and information service for people in Scotland. You can contact them by:

Phone at 08454 24 24 24 or online at *www.nhs24.com*

Contact details for Welsh local health boards and the Health Service Ombudsman of Wales are:

To find contact details for your local health board:
look in the phone book under "health services"
or look online at www.wales.nhs.uk

Health Service Ombudsman for Wales
Office of the Health Service Ombudsman for Wales
5th Floor, Capital Tower, Greyfriars Road
CARDIFF, CF10 3AG
Phone: 029 2039 4621
Fax: 029 2022 6909
www.ombudsman.org.uk

NHS Direct Wales

HS Direct Wales (Galw Iechyd Cymru) is the NHS Direct service for people in Wales. It provides information in English and Welsh. You can contact them by phone at 0845 4647 or online at *www. nhsdirect.wales.nhs.uk.*

PART SEVEN

FREE AUDIO, CONTACTS AND GLOSSARY

33

FREE AUDIO RECORDING AND SPECIAL REPORT

"Making the Perfect Treatment Choice"

Are you confused about all your treatment choices, or concerned about making the wrong treatment decision?

If so you are not alone—many people leave the dentist feeling more confused about their choices than before they went in.

No dentist will tell you what you must do, they can only advise you what you can do! So, how do you use their advice to make the best decision for you?

Find out how to choose the perfect treatment for you and much more, for whatever type of care you are looking for.

Download Free Recording and Special Report NOW at

www.MyPerfectDentist.com

34
USEFUL CONTACTS

American Academy of Cosmetic Dentistry—AACD
www.aacd.com
Tel: 001 8005439220

Association of Dental Implantology—ADI
www.adi.org.co.uk
98 South Warpole Way
London
SW14 8ND
Tel: 0208 4875555

British Academy of Aesthetic Dentistry—BAAD
www.baad.org.uk

British Academy of Cosmetic Dentistry—BACD
www.bacd.com
29 Harley Street
London W1G 9QR
Tel: +44 20 7612 4166

British Association of Oral Surgeons
www.baos.org.uk

British Dental Association—BDA
www.bda.org
64 Wimpole Street,
London
W1G8YS
Tel: 020 7935 0875

British Endodontic Society
www.BritishEndodonticSociety.org.uk.
PO Box 707
Gerrards Cross
Bucks
SL9 0XS
Tel/Fax 01494 581542

British Orthodontic Society
www.bos.org.uk
12 Bridewell Place,
London EC4V 6AP
Tel: 020 7353 8680

British Society of Occlusal Studies—BSOS
www.bsos.org.uk

British Society of Paediatric Dentistry
www.bspd.co.uk

British Society of Periodontology
www.bsperio.org.uk
PO BOX 334
LEEDS
LS19 9FJ
Tel/Fax 0844 335 1915

British Society for the Study of Prosthodontics
www.bsspd.org

Cosmetic Dentistry Guide
www.CosmeticDentistryGuide.com

Dental Complaints Service
www.dentalcomplaints.org.uk
The Dental Complaints Service
The Lansdowne Building
2 Lansdowne Road
Croydon
CR9 2ER
TEL: 08456 120 540

Dental Health Foundation— British Dental Health Foundation/ International Dental Health Foundation
www.DentalHealth.org.uk
Smile House
2 East Union Street
Rugby
Warwickshire
CV22 6AJ
United Kingdom
Email: mail@dentalhealth.org
Dental Helpline: 0845 063 1188
(local call rate in the UK)
Fax: +44 (0) 870 770 4010

General Dental Council—GDC
www.gdc-uk.org
General Dental Council
37 Wimpole Street

London
W1G 8DQ
Tel: 0845 222 4141 (UK local rate)
or 020 7887 3800
From abroad: +44 20 7887 3800
Fax: +44 (0) 20 7224 3294
The GDC also offers a "typetalk" facility for customers with impaired hearing. This can be accessed by calling 18001 0845 222 4141 on your typetalk/minicom handset.

I Want Great Care—
Web-based ratings site
www.IWantGreatCare.org

MyPerfect Dentist
www.MyPerfectDentist.com

Contact Details for Dental Complaints:

Citizens Advice Bureau
Your local Citizens Advice Bureau can be a great source of advice and support if you want to complain about the NHS, social services, or local authorities. You can find your local Citizens Advice Bureau online for England, Wales, and Northern Ireland at www.citizensadvice.org.uk. For Scotland, go to *www.cas.org.uk*.

Dental Complaints Service
www.dentalcomplaints.org.uk
The Dental Complaints Service
The Lansdowne Building
2 Lansdowne Road
Croydon
CR9 2ER
TEL: 08456 120 540

England

Independent Complaints Advocacy Service

The Independent Complaints Advocacy Service (ICAS) is a national service that supports people who wish to make a complaint about their NHS care or treatment. Contact your local ICAS office through the hospital manager or PALS, or by calling the following numbers:
London: 0845 120 3784
South East: 0845 600 8616
Bedfordshire and Hertfordshire: 0845 456 1082
Cambridgeshire, Norfolk and Suffolk: 0845 456 1084
Essex: 0845 456 1083
South West: 0845 120 3782
West Midlands: 0845 120 3748
East Midlands: 0845 650 0088
North East: 0845 120 3732
North West: 0845 120 3735
Yorkshire and Humberside: 0845 120 3734

NHS Complaints Service (England)
www.nhs.uk

NHS Direct England
NHS Direct can advise on NHS complaints. Call 0845 4647.

Northern Ireland

Northern Ireland Health and Social Care Board
Call your local care board at 0800 665544 or online at *www.n-i.nhs.uk*.

Alternatively, contact the central office at:
12-22 Linenhall Street
Belfast,
BT2 8BS
028 9043 4004

Northern Ireland Ombudsman
33 Wellington Place
Belfast
BT1 6HN
www.ni-ombudsman.org.uk

Scotland

Scottish Local Health Boards
To find contact details for your local NHS board:
look in the phone book under "health services"
call the NHS Helpline on 0800 22 44 88 (textphone 18001 0800 22 44 88), or look online at
www.hris.org.uk **or**
www.show.scot.nhs.uk/organisations/orgindex.htm

Scottish Public Services Ombudsman
The Scottish Public Services Ombudsman
Freepost EH641
Edinburgh
EH3 0BR
Phone: 0800 377 7330
Fax: 0800 377 7331
Text message: 07900 494 372
E-mail: ask@spso.org.uk
Website: *www.spso.org.uk*

Scotland—NHS 24

NHS 24 is a twenty-four-hour telephone health advice and information service for people in Scotland. You can contact them by phone at 08454 24 24 24 or online at *www.nhs24.com*.

Wales

Welsh Local Health Boards

To find contact details for your local health board:
look in the phone book under "health services"
or look online at *www.wales.nhs.uk*

Health Service Ombudsman of Wales

Office of the Health Service Ombudsman for Wales
5th Floor, Capital Tower
Greyfriars Road
CARDIFF
CF10 3AG
Phone: 029 2039 4621
Fax: 029 2022 6909
www.ombudsman.org.uk

NHS Direct Wales

NHS Direct Wales (Galw Iechyd Cymru) is the NHS Direct service for people in Wales. It provides information in English and Welsh. You can contact them by phone at 0845 4647 or online at *www. nhsdirect.wales.nhs.uk*.

35
GLOSSARY OF TERMS

Abutment — A tooth or implant used to support a prosthesis. A crown unit used as part of a fixed bridge.

Abscess — A localized inflammation due to a collection of pus in the bone or soft tissue, usually caused by an infection.

Amalgam — A dental filling material, composed of mercury and other minerals, used to fill decayed teeth.

Anaesthetic — A class of drugs that eliminates or reduces pain. See local anaesthetic.

Anterior — Refers to the teeth and tissues located towards the front of the mouth (upper or lower incisors and canines).

Apex — The tip end of a root.

Apexification — A method of inducing apical closure, or the continual apical development of the root of an incompletely formed tooth, in which the pulp is no longer vital.

Autoclave — A medical autoclave is a device that uses steam to sterilize equipment.

Bicuspid — A two-cuspid tooth found between the molar and the cuspid also known as an eye tooth or canine tooth.

Biopsy — A process of removing tissue to determine the existence of pathology.

Bitewing X-ray — Radiograph taken of the crowns of teeth to check for decay (caries).

Bonding — A process to chemically etch the tooth's enamel to better attach (bond) composite filling material, veneers or plastic/acrylic.

Bone loss — The breakdown and loss of the bone that supports the teeth, usually caused by infection or long-term occlusal (chewing areas of the teeth) stress.

Bridge— A fixed prosthetic replacement of one or more missing teeth, cemented or attached to the abutment teeth or implant abutments adjacent to the space.

Bruxism — The involuntary clenching or grinding of the teeth.

Calculus — The hard deposit of mineralized plaque that forms on the crown and/or root of the tooth. Also referred to as tartar.

Canine tooth — The second tooth from the big front tooth, commonly called the eye tooth.

Cantilever Extension — Part of a fixed prosthesis that is supported at one end only.

Cap — Another term for crown; usually referring to a crown for a front tooth.

Caries — The correct technical term for decay, which is the progressive breaking down or dissolving of tooth structure caused by the acid produced when bacteria digest sugars.

Cavity — A layman's term for decay. Also, the dental term for the hole that is left after the decay has been removed.

Cement — A special type of glue used to hold a crown in its place. It also acts as an insulator to protect the tooth's nerve.

Cementum — The very thin, bonelike structure that covers the root of the tooth.

Clenching — The forceful holding together of the upper and lower teeth, which places stress on the ligaments that hold the teeth to the jawbone, and the lower jaw to the skull.

Complex rehabilitation — The extensive dental restoration involving multiple units of crown and/or bridge in the same treatment plan. Using full crowns and/or fixed bridges, which are cemented in place, that your dentist will use to rebuild natural teeth fill in spaces where teeth are missing and establish conditions which allow each tooth to function in harmony with the occlusion (bite).

Composite — A tooth-coloured restoration (filling) made of plastic resin or porcelain.

Consultation — A diagnostic service provided by a dentist other than the treating dentist.

Cosmetic dentistry — Any dental treatment or repair that is solely rendered to improve the appearance of the teeth or mouth.

Crown — The portion of a tooth that is covered by enamel. Also a dental restoration that covers the entire tooth and restores it to its original shape.

Crown lengthening — A surgical procedure exposing more of the tooth for restorative purposes.

Curettage — A deep scaling of that portion of the tooth below the gum line. Purpose is to reduce bacterial load, remove calculus and infected gum tissue.

Cuspid — See canine tooth.

Cusp(s) — The protruding portion(s) of a tooth's chewing surface.

Decay — See caries.

Deciduous — See primary teeth.

Dental Floss — A thin, nylon string, waxed or unwaxed, that is inserted between the teeth and under the gums to remove food and plaque.

Dental Hygienist — A dental professional specialising in the prevention and treatment of gum diseases. She/he acts as the patient's guide in establishing a proper oral hygiene program, along with removing plaque and/or calculus from the crown and roots of teeth.

Dentine — The part of the tooth that is under both the enamel which covers the crown and the cementum which covers the root.

Dentition — The teeth in the dental arch.

Denture — A removable appliance used to replace teeth. A complete denture replaces all of the upper teeth and/or all the lower teeth.

Diastema — A space, such as one between two adjacent teeth in the same dental arch.

Distal — Farther from any part of reference.

Direct pulp cap — The procedure in which the exposed pulp is covered with a dressing or cement that protects the pulp and promotes healing and repair.

Dry socket (osteitis) — A localized inflammation of the tooth socket following an extraction due to infection of a blood clot.

Enamel — The hard, calcified (mineralized) portion of the tooth which covers the crown. Enamel is the hardest substance in the body.

Endodontics — The dental specialty that deals with injuries to or diseases of the pulp, or nerve, of the tooth.

Endodontist — A dentist who deals with the cause, prevention, diagnosis, and treatment or injuries and diseases that affect the dental pulp, tooth root and periapical tissue.

Extraction — The removal of a tooth.

Excision — Surgical removal of bone or tissue.

Extraoral — Pertaining to the outside of the mouth.

Facial — Pertaining to or toward the face (Buccal, Labial).

Filling — Material used to fill cavity or replace part of a tooth. Often referred to as a restoration.

Fissure — A deep ditch or cleft in the surface of the teeth.

Fissure sealant — A plastic coating bonded to the tooth surface with the intention of sealing a fissure against decay causing bacteria

Floss — See dental floss.

Fluoride — A chemical compound used to prevent dental decay, utilized in fluoridated water systems and/or applied directly to the teeth.

Frenum — Muscle fibres covered by a mucus membrane that attaches the check, lips and/or tongue to associated dental mucous membrane.

Frenectomy — The removal of a frenum.

Gingiva — The soft tissue that covers the jawbone. Also referred to as the gums.

Gingivectomy — A surgical removal of the gingiva (gum tissue).

Gingivitis — An inflammation or infection of the gingiva; the initial stage of gum disease.

Graft — A piece of tissue or synthetic material placed in contact with tissue to repair a defect or supplement a deficiency.

Gum — See gingivitis.

Gum Disease — See periodontal disease.

Gum-lift — The surgical repositioning of the visible gum line around the teeth to a higher level. This may involve surgical repositioning of the gum, underlying jawbone or combination of the two.

Immediate denture — A denture constructed for immediate placement after removal of the remaining teeth.

Impacted tooth — An un-erupted or partially erupted tooth that is positioned against another tooth, bone or soft tissue so that total eruption is unlikely.

Implant — An artificial device, usually made of Titanium metal alloy or ceramic material, that is implanted within the jawbone as a means to attach an artificial crown, denture or bridge.

Incipient — Dental caries in an early stage of development, usually not requiring immediate restorations.

Incisal — Pertaining to the cutting edges of incisor and canine teeth.

Indirect pulp cap — A procedure in which the nearly exposed pulp is covered with a protective dressing to protect the pulp from additional injury and to promote healing and repair via formation of secondary dentin.

Inlay — A cast gold filling that is used to replace part of the tooth.

Interproximal — The area between two adjacent teeth.

Intraoral — The inside of a mouth.

Labial — The area pertaining to or around the lip.

Lingual — The area pertaining to or around the tongue.

Local Anaesthetic — The injection given in the mouth to numb the areas where a tooth or area needs a dental procedure. Often referred to as Lignocaine.

Malocclusion — The improper alignment of biting or chewing surfaces of upper and lower teeth.

Mandible — The lower jaw.

Maryland bridge — The trade name that becomes synonymous with any resin bonded fixed partial denture (bridge).

Mastication — The act of chewing.

Maxilla — The upper jaw.

Mesial — Toward or situated in the middle.

Molars — The broad, multicusped back teeth, used for grinding food; they are considered the largest teeth in the mouth. In adults there are a total of twelve molars (including the four wisdom teeth, or third molars), three on each side of the upper and lower jaws.

Nitrous oxide — A controlled mixture of nitrogen and oxygen gases (N2O) that is inhaled by the patient in order to decrease sensitivity to pain. Also referred to as laughing gas.

Occlusal X-ray — An intraoral X-ray taken with the film held between the teeth in biting position.

Occlusal surface — The chewing surface of the back teeth.

Occlusion — Any contact between biting or chewing surfaces of upper and lower teeth.

Onlay — A cast gold or porcelain filling that covers one or all of the tooth's cusps.

Oral surgery — The removal of teeth and the repair and treatment of other oral problems, such as tumours and fractures.

Orthodontics — A specialised branch of dentistry that corrects malocclusion and restores the teeth to proper alignment and function. There are several different types of appliances used in orthodontics, one of which is commonly referred to as braces.

Overbite — A condition in which the upper teeth excessively overlap the lower teeth when the jaw is closed.

Overjet — A condition in which the upper teeth excessively protrude the lower teeth when the jaw is closed.

Palate — The hard and soft tissues forming the roof of the mouth.

Palliative — Treatment that relieves pain but is *not* curative.

Partial denture — A removable appliance used to replace one or more lost teeth.

Paediatric dentistry — The specialised branch of dentistry that deals solely with treating children's dental disease.

Periapical — The area that surrounds the tip of a tooth's root.

Pericoronitis — An inflammation of the gum tissue around the crown of a tooth, usually the third molar.

Periodontal — Relating to the tissue and bone that supports the tooth (from *peri*, meaning 'around,' and *dont* meaning 'tooth').

Periodontal disease — The inflammation and infection of the gums, ligaments, bone, and other tissues surrounding the teeth.

Periodontal pocket — An abnormal deepening of the gingival crevice. It is caused when disease and infection destroy the ligament that attaches the gum to the tooth and the underlying bone.

Periodontics — The area of dentistry concerned with the diagnosis, prevention and treatment of periodontal disease.

Periodontist. — The dental specialty that deals with and treats the gum tissue and bone that supports the teeth.

Periodontitis — Inflammation of the supporting structures of the tooth, including the gum, the periodontal ligament, and the jawbone.

Periradicular — The area which surrounds a portion of the root of the tooth.

Permanent teeth — The thirty-two adult teeth that replace the baby, or primary, teeth. Also known as secondary teeth.

Pit — A recessed area found on the surface of a tooth, usually where the grooves of the tooth meet.

Plaque — A film of sticky material containing saliva, food particles and bacteria that attaches to the tooth surface both above and below the gum line. When left on the tooth it can promote gum disease and decay.

Pontic — An artificial tooth used in a bridge to replace a missing tooth.

Post and core — An elongated metallic projection fitted and cemented within the prepared root canal, serving to strengthen and retain restorative material and/or a crown restoration.

Premolar — Another name for bicuspid.

Preventative dentistry — Education and treatment devoted to and concerned with preventing the development of dental diseases.

Preventative treatment — Any action taken by the patient, assisted by the dentist or hygienist, that serves to prevent dental or other disease. Sealants, cleanings and space maintainers are examples of preventative treatment.

Primary teeth — The first set of teeth that humans get, lasting until the permanent teeth come in. Also referred to as baby or deciduous teeth.

Prophylaxis — The scaling and polishing procedure performed to remove calculus, plaque and stains from the crowns of the teeth.

Prosthesis (dental) — Any device or appliance replacing one or more missing teeth.

Prosthodontics — The dental specialty dealing with the replacement of missing teeth and other oral structures.

Pulp — The hollow chamber inside the crown of the tooth that contains its nerves and blood vessels.

Pulpotomy — The removal of a portion of the tooth's pulp.

Quadrant — The dental term for the division of the jaws onto four parts, beginning at the midline of the arch and extending towards the last tooth in the back of the mouth. There are four quadrants in the mouth; each quadrant generally contains five to eight teeth.

Receded gums — A condition characterised by the abnormal loss of gum tissue due to infection or bone loss.

Referral — When a dental patient is sent to another dentist, usually a specialist, for treatment or consultation.

Reline — The process of resurfacing the tissue side of a denture with a base material.

Replantation — The return of a tooth to its socket.

Resorption — The breakdown and assimilation of the bone that supports the tooth; i.e., bone loss.

Restoration — Any material or devise used to replace lost tooth structure (filling, crown) or to replace a lost tooth or teeth (bridge, dentures, complete or partial).

Retainer — A removable dental appliance, usually used in orthodontics, that maintains space between teeth or holds teeth in a fixed position until the bone solidifies around them.

Root — The part of the tooth below the crown, normally encased in the jawbone. It is made up of dentine, includes the root canal, and is covered by cementum.

Root Canal — The hollow part of the tooth's root. It runs from the tip of the root into the pulp.

Root canal therapy — The process of treating disease or inflammation of the pulp or root canal. This involves removing the pulp and root's nerve(s) and filling the canal(s) with an appropriate material to permanently seal it.

Root planning — The process of scaling and planning exposed root surfaces to remove all calculus, plaque and infected tissue.

Scaling — A procedure used to remove plaque, calculus and stains from the teeth.

Sealant — A composite material used to seal the decay-prone pits, fissures and grooves of teeth to prevent decay.

Six-year molar — The first permanent tooth to erupt, usually between the ages of five and six.

Socket — The hole in the jawbone into which the tooth fits.

Space maintainer — A dental appliance that fills the space of a lost tooth or teeth and prevents the other teeth from moving into the space. Used especially in orthodontic treatment.

Subgingival scaling — The removal of calculus and plaque found on the tooth below the gum line.

Supra gingival scaling — The removal of calculus and plaque found on the tooth above the gum line.

Systemic — Relating to the whole body.

Tartar — See calculus.

Temporomandibular joint (TMJ) — The connecting hinge mechanism between the lower jaw and the base of the skull.

Third molar — The last of the three molar teeth, also called wisdom teeth. There are four third molars—two in the lower jaw, two in the upper jaw—on each side.

Torus — A bony elevation of normal bone. Usually seen on the upper palate behind the front teeth or under the tongue inside the lower jaw.

Treatment plan — A list of work that the dentist proposes to perform on a dental patient based on the results of the radiographs, examination and diagnosis. Often more than one treatment plan is presented.

Veneer — An artificial restorative material, usually plastic, composite or porcelain, that is used to provide an aesthetic covering over the visible surface of a tooth. Most often used on front teeth.

Wisdom teeth — See third molar.

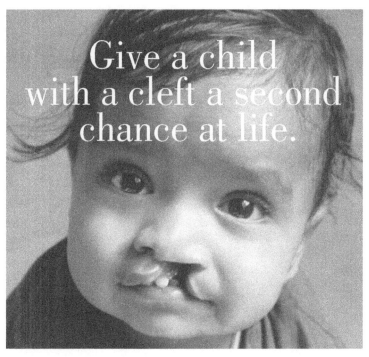

Give a child with a cleft a second chance at life.

Shiva was born with a severe cleft lip and palate in a very poor, rural area of Northern India. Like millions of children born with clefts in the developing world, Shiva faced a life of discrimination, stigma and physical pain. He may have been excluded from school and had to suffer the cruel taunts of people who believed his cleft was the result of a 'curse'.

Since Smile Train operated when he was so young, Shiva was saved from many years of pain and heartbreak. And he will never develop the kind of speech impediment that is often impossible to correct in children who have their clefts repaired much later in life. He may never know how lucky he is.

Cleft surgery for a child like Shiva costs only around £150 and can take as little as 45 minutes. Please send a donation today and give a child like Shiva not only a new smile, but a second chance at life.

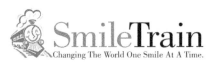

SmileTrain
Changing The World One Smile At A Time.

Donate online: www.smiletrain.org.uk
OR call: 0870 127 6269

© 2010 The Smile Train.

www.ingramcontent.com/pod-product-compliance
Lightning Source LLC
Jackson TN
JSHW020020141224
75386JS00025B/623

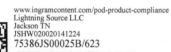